THE
OXYGEN
CURE

THE

OXYGEN CURE

A Complete Guide to Hyperbaric Oxygen Therapy

William S. Maxfield, MD, and Jodie Gould

Humanix Books

The Oxygen Cure
Copyright © 2017 by Humanix Books
All rights reserved

Humanix Books, P.O. Box 20989, West Palm Beach, FL 33416, USA
www.humanixbooks.com | info@humanixbooks.com

Library of Congress Cataloging-in-Publication Data

Names: Maxfield, William S., author.
Title: The oxygen cure : a complete guide to hyperbaric oxygen therapy /
Dr. William S. Maxfield.
Description: West Palm Beach, FL : Humanix Books, [2016] | Includes index.
Identifiers: LCCN 2016037589 (print) | LCCN 2016038341 (ebook) |
ISBN 9781630060510 (paperback) | ISBN 9781630060527 (E-book) | ISBN
9781630060527 (e-book)
Subjects: LCSH: Hyperbaric oxygenation. | BISAC: HEALTH & FITNESS /
Alternative Therapies. | HEALTH & FITNESS / Diseases / General. | HEALTH &
FITNESS / Pain Management.
Classification: LCC RM666.O83 M39 2016 (print) | LCC RM666.O83 (ebook) |
DDC 615.8/36—dc23
LC record available at https://lccn.loc.gov/2016037589

Cover Design: Tom Lau
Interior Design: Scribe Inc.

Humanix Books is a division of Humanix Publishing, LLC. Its trademark,
consisting of the words "Humanix" is registered in the Patent and Trademark
Office and in other countries.

Disclaimer: The information presented in this book is meant to be used for
general resource purposes only; it is not intended as specific medical advice
for any individual and should not substitute medical advice from a healthcare
professional. If you have (or think you may have) a medical problem, speak to
your doctor or healthcare practitioner immediately about your risk and possible
treatments. Do not engage in any therapy or treatment without consulting a
medical professional.

ISBN: 978-1-63006-051-0 (Trade Paper)
ISBN: 978-1-63006-052-7 (E-book)

Printed in the United States of America
10 9 8 7 6 5 4 3 2 1

CONTENTS

PREFACE

For more than 25 years, I've worked as a specialist in hyperbaric oxygen therapy (HBOT), a medical procedure in which you enter an enclosed body chamber to breathe pure oxygen at air pressure levels that are higher than what we naturally inhale. You do not need a medical degree to understand how HBOT works. Did you know that there is 21 percent oxygen in the air that we breathe? Simply put, HBOT works by having patients breathe 100 percent oxygen in a pressurized, closed environment. The lungs transfer this oxygen to the red blood cells (more on those later) and push oxygen into the fluid of the blood. The oxygen-filled cells are then carried around the body by the plasma (fluid), which travels through the blood vessels. HBOT uses oxygen to treat tissues in the body that have been damaged by oxygen deprivation.

What happens next is nothing short of miraculous. By giving our bodies these infusions of oxygen where we need them most (at various levels and frequencies), we can heal wounds and burns, restore lost cognitive function, treat cancer patients suffering from chemotherapy side effects, and, at times, help myriad illnesses and diseases go into remission. HBOT is a holistic treatment that targets the underlying disease or condition, not just the symptoms.

As a board-certified physician in hyperbaric medicine, radiology, and nuclear medicine, I've seen thousands of seemingly "hopeless cases" transformed by this natural healing process. I'm currently a HBOT consultant based in Odessa, Florida, where I treat a wide range of medical conditions, including dementia, stroke, heart ailments, migraines, asthma, emphysema, arthritis, multiple sclerosis, HIV/AIDS, cerebral palsy, and posttraumatic stress disorder (PTSD).

My colleagues and I have saved countless fingers, toes, legs, and hands from amputation. We've helped the bedridden to walk, the mute to talk, and the deaf to hear, and the near blind to see. "Hold on a minute," you say. "Is Dr. Maxfield a doctor or a faith healer? Why should I trust a treatment that hasn't been entirely embraced by the American Medical Association and only approved for 14 indications by the Food and Drug Administration (FDA)?" All I can tell you is that medicine isn't perfect and it continues to make advances and to evolve. If you are old enough, you might remember a time when smoking cigarettes was not considered hazardous to your health by the surgeon general. And what once seemed more like science fiction than real science (transplants, preventive vaccines, laser surgery) is now taken for granted. The same is the case for HBOT, which, although misunderstood by many in traditional medicine and still the best-kept medical secret, is rapidly becoming a widely accepted as a scientifically proven medical alternative to drug therapy and invasive surgeries. I will explain why this proven therapy has been kept under wraps.

When people think of HBOT, they might picture Michael Jackson sleeping in an oxygen chamber in search of eternal youth. What you might not know is that he discovered HBOT at a hospital while recovering from a burn he received while filming a commercial. As it turns out, not only is hyperbaric oxygen therapy an approved and excellent treatment for burns, it has also been found to help certain conditions associated with aging, such as osteoporosis, arthritis, dementia, poor eyesight, and even wrinkles. It is currently most often used for traumatic brain injuries and healing wounds.

While HBOT sounds breathtakingly simple, keep in mind that it is a medical procedure that should be supervised and administered (at least in the beginning of treatment) by a trained and certified oxygen therapy clinician. The correct dose of HBOT varies depending on each person's condition. Patients are exposed to increased levels of oxygen delivered over a period of time. Doctors like me, and other experts included in this book who are trained in HBOT, decide on a patient's protocol based on their experience, research, and the patient's scan results.

The good news for those who have tried and failed with other treatments, including surgeries or medications, or have been told by traditional physicians that HBOT is quackery—or worse, harmful—there are more and more studies and clinical trials being done every year that verify hyperbaric oxygen therapy's remarkable healing properties and even curative benefits for a variety of common conditions and life-threatening diseases. HBOT has being widely used in other countries such as Russia, China, Cuba, Canada, England, Israel, and parts of South America for decades with enormous success.

My Journey to HBOT and Alternative Medicine

I come from a family of physicians, including my father and my two brothers, who were all doctors. My father, who was a general practitioner, was a believer in alternative medicine— and many years ahead of his time—during the early 20th century. He was the first to use an X-ray machine in east Texas in 1903. I still have a photo of the machine, which was operated with a hand-crank. In the picture, there are electrical wires on the ceiling and the wall coming to the machine. My father had added an electric motor, and a year later, that same machine was powered by electricity. My dad worked in an East Texas town that had salt mines, so many of his patients would come in with work-related fractures. My dad recognized the value that an X-ray machine provided by helping him diagnosis his patients' injuries.

My father preferred natural remedies that treated the underlying disease rather than the symptoms, which is what traditional medicine tends to do. He was so ahead of his time that he understood the connection between lifestyle and health, and he would frequently advise his patients to keep their weight down by eating nutritionally balanced foods and exercising. I remember him forbidding my siblings and me from eating ice cream, not because of the dangers of sugar, but because he thought it was too cold. His theory turned out not to be scientifically sound, but, conversely, research now shows the risks of contracting esophageal cancer from drinking beverages, such as coffee, that are too hot.

My love of medicine and holistic healing, which I inherited from my father, continued when I was at Baylor College of Medicine in Houston, Texas, during the '50s. On my first day, the dean gave a welcome lecture to the med students telling us, "Unfortunately, half of what you are going to learn in the next four years is not going to be true; it's up to you to figure out which half is right and which half is wrong."

This is the approach that I have carried with me throughout my career. I was first introduced to hyperbaric oxygen in the navy as part of the decontamination team. It was there that I learned how HBOT helps cure "the bends" (also known as Caisson disease or decompression sickness), a condition that causes brain damage in divers when a change in pressure produces air bubbles in the vascular system.

I decided to further explore other uses for HBOT by looking at the data from Europe, where they were experimenting with HBOT as an adjunct to cancer treatment. When using radiation therapy, researchers discovered that normal cells would increase after HBOT. They experimented by giving patients hyperbaric therapy first, waiting a period of time, then doing radiation, which brought the cancer cells down to a normal level.

I also served as chief of the Radioisotope Laboratory at the US Naval Hospital in Bethesda, Maryland, and was part of plutonium decontamination team. Later, as chief of radiation therapy at the Ochsner Clinic and Foundation Hospital in New Orleans, I included a hyperbaric unit in the new radiation therapy department. By the early '80s, I had established the Gulf South Radiation Center in Largo, Florida, the first HBOT facility in the area. Since then, I have treated hundreds of wounded warriors who returned home from battle with brain traumas, PTSD, and severe blast injuries, many of whom were in tremendous pain or suicidal. I am proud to play a part in restoring these heroes to their former lives by preventing the loss of a leg or by helping them battle debilitating depression.

While I was at Johns Hopkins School of Medicine, Tulane University School of Medicine, and Louisiana State University—all fine institutions—HBOT was not a part of the curriculum. But it is my fervent hope that the increased awareness of hyperbaric oxygen therapy will allow future generations of medical students to learn about its uses and be able to recommend HBOT in whatever specialty they go on to practice. To those in the health care community who care more about profits than patients, I say, when correctly applied, HBOT not only benefits sick people, it can reduce our country's staggeringly high medical costs.

To readers of this book who might be suffering or know someone who is, I will explain what oxygen therapy can do for you or your loved ones. I will debunk many of the myths about HBOT, including the belief that it belongs on the fringes of medicine. There have been many attempts to eliminate the use of hyperbaric oxygen therapy, including one physician who built a hyperbaric chamber in the '30s that was shut down by the American Medical Association. The fight for acceptance and for increased insurance coverage continues today, despite the amazing results from studies and the personal stories that you will read about in this book.

The Oxygen Cure is born of my desire and passion to educate people—believers and skeptics—about the benefits of this simple yet extraordinary treatment. To that end, I have included the testimonies of some of the best practitioners in the field in this book as well as the heart-wrenching and heart-warming stories of people who have received HBOT, which were given willingly and enthusiastically because they too have a shared passion to let the world know about how this therapy that has changed their lives. Collectively we share first-hand experiences with HBOT. But, anecdotal evidence aside, it is important to emphasize again that this therapy has been scientifically tested and is proven to work. HBOT will only be widely accepted by the mainstream medical community if enough people ask or *demand* that they receive this life-changing treatment! My advice is to ask your doctor about hyperbaric therapy. If he or she is either unfamiliar with it, unwilling to discuss it, or dismissive, find another doctor or consult the resource section at the end of this book for referrals to HBOT clinics, hospitals, and practitioners near you.

I will tell you who the best candidates are for treatment, answer the most frequently asked questions about HBOT, and give you additional healing and lifestyle tips for many of the conditions described in this book. If you are sick, in pain, or know someone who is, you have the right to know about all the available options that technology and medicine has to offer. *The Oxygen Cure* will act as your guide to better health and well-being through hyperbaric oxygen therapy.

—William S. Maxfield, MD, FACNM

1

WHAT IS HYPERBARIC OXYGEN THERAPY?

· ·

Hyperbaric oxygen is just too simple for most doctors to understand; they have forgotten their basic gas laws of physics.

—Edward Teller, Nobel Prize–winning physicist

I met Dr. Edward Teller, the Nobel Prize–winning physicist who developed the technology that produced the hydrogen bomb, while working with the Atomic Energy Commission and NASA. We became lifelong friends, and I became one of his family's consulting physicians. Teller and his wife,

Missy, eventually moved to California, where he taught at Stanford University. It was there that Missy first used hyperbaric therapy. After being diagnosed with chronic obstructive pulmonary disease (COPD) when she was in her 70s, the pulmonologist at Stanford gave her only a few months to live. Hyperbaric oxygen therapy was not being practiced in California at the time, so I gave Dr. Richard Neubauer, a pioneer in the field of HBOT and a former colleague of mine, Missy's records to review. Dr. Neubauer famously coined the term "idling neuron" in his theory about the ability of injured brain cells to wake up or come back to life using hyperbaric oxygen.

Dr. Neubauer and I suggested that the Tellers get a home oxygen chamber, and we supervised her treatments. After six weeks of HBOT, Missy made a full recovery. She got five more productive years and eventually died from a cerebral vascular accident, completely unrelated to her emphysema.

After seeing how HBOT helped save his wife, Teller became an advocate. He even used it himself after suffering a stroke at the age of 84, leaving him mentally impaired and unable to travel on his own. After receiving HBOT treatments, his cognitive function returned and he was able return to work and travel by himself. Dr. Teller's status as a brilliant physicist and research scientist helped legitimize this otherwise overlooked form of medicine. He even spoke about HBOT at the American College of Hyperbaric Medicine. He is said to have spent an hour a day in his home chamber until his death from a massive stroke at the age of

95. Although HBOT wasn't able to save him after his second stroke, his continued use of hyperbaric oxygen helped keep his mind sharp and his body active until the very end.

But before I tell you more about the uses for hyperbaric oxygen therapy and its success stories, I want to explain exactly what it is and how it works. Most people understand that oxygen is a natural, life-sustaining substance. HBOT, a noninvasive, nonmedicinal procedure, harnesses the healing power of oxygen by administering it to patients who are inside a special hyperbaric chamber using an air compressor or oxygen tank. It works on a cellular level by being absorbed into tissues in the body that are oxygen deprived so they can heal or keep from dying out.

Dr. Paul G. Harch, a New Orleans–based hyperbaric and emergency medicine physician and president of the International Hyperbaric Medical Association, explains it this way: "When oxygen is under pressure, it has drug-like effects on the DNA and other components of each cell, bringing about permanent changes in the cell and surrounding tissue. In this way HBOT is one of the most effective gene therapies. Over the years of experimenting with HBOT, we've discovered that the secret to its success is its cumulative effect, meaning that after 25 to 40 treatments, the body's tissues can be *permanently* changed."

Some of Dr. Harch's patients have spoken to us about their recovery, and he documents the latest groundbreaking treatments for hyperbaric oxygen in his own book, *The Oxygen Revolution*, written with Virginia McCullough. His clinic is one of the finest in the country. Other specialists in hyperbaric therapy and their patients are also included in this book, and I'm grateful for their work and their contributions. Before we move on the case stories and conditions, here are some commonly asked questions that most people have when considering HBOT treatments.

How Is HBOT Done?

HBOT is done inside a pressurized oxygen chamber during what is called a "dive," a term borrowed from scuba diving. When given 100 percent oxygen, an injury site absorbs the correct healing dose. HBOT practitioners commonly use enriched oxygen, an oxygen concentrator, or an oxygen generator. The oxygen is infused into the numerous types of liquids in the body, such as blood, plasma, and cerebral fluids. This oxygen uptake will remain in the body for a period of time after treatment. According to the gas laws of physics, more gas is dissolved in a liquid by increasing the pressure of the gas.

How Long Are HBOT Sessions, and How Many Treatments Do People Typically Get?

The length of treatments depends on the doctor's particular protocol for that individual. Every person and every condition is unique. Hyperbaric treatments may require a one-hour or two-hour session. Some treatment programs might require three treatments a week for several weeks or more. In severe cases, people can have hundreds of sessions and continue with maintenance throughout their lifetime. Every patient's protocol is different.

Just Breathe

The air we breathe is made up of 79% nitrogen, 20.9% oxygen, and 0.1% carbon dioxide and all other gases. In one hour, humans can inhale 2.4 pounds of oxygen! The air pressure at sea level is called 1 atmosphere absolute (ATA). When a scuba diver is at a depth of 10 meters, the total absolute pressure on the diver is 2 ATA. When we breathe, red blood cells instantly fill with oxygen and any additional oxygen dissolves directly into the blood fluid.[1]

When Was HBOT First Used?

Oxygen therapy was believed to be first used in 1664 by an Englishman named N. Henshaw who built a metal chamber to which he attached two large bellows that pushed oxygen into the chamber. This was the first pressurized therapy machine. It is not known if Henshaw was a doctor or a pastor (or both), but either way, his treatments were never adopted in medical circles. Meanwhile, across the channel in France, there was a trend afoot called "air baths," which, like water spas, were thought to improve overall health. People would soak in these pressure baths for hours. The baths eventually closed when people stayed beyond the decompression limits and began feeling sick.

Oxygen therapy was resurrected in the United States during the 1918 Spanish flu epidemic, when Dr. Orval Cunningham of the University of Kansas noticed that sick people fared better at higher elevations than those who were at sea level. He eventually built the Cunningham Sanitarium, a five-story structure designed to maintain a pressurized atmosphere. This hospital was the first to conduct oxygen therapy on a large scale.

Dr. Cunningham was convinced that the higher air pressure introduced an increased amount of oxygen into the body, which helped patients with lung disease. Because lungs are one of the main organs affected by influenza viruses, word, like the virus, soon spread about Dr. Cunningham's discovery. But despite his growing reputation in the field of hyperbaric medicine, once again colleagues in mainstream medicine discredited his work and writings.

In the 1800s, a French physician named V. T. Junod theorized that compressed air increased blood flow to the brain and other organs. His theory turned out to be correct as well, and it is the basis for modern HBOT treatments that offer repeated use of hyperbaric oxygen to promote new blood vessel growth. Experiments were done with pressurized air, but researchers still did not understand why or how hyperbaric oxygen worked.

Hyperbaric oxygen therapy remained on the fringes of health care until the '50s, when doctors in the Netherlands discovered that HBOT could treat a life-threatening infection like gas gangrene, which can occur in those with severe wounds. Physicians there found that oxygen kills the anaerobic (non-oxygen-using) bacteria that cause the infection. It was during this experiment in the Holland that scientists proved that pigs could survive in a hyperbaric chamber without blood. Doctors removed all the pigs' blood and replaced it with saline before giving them pure oxygen. (This study eventually led to the use of HBOT for pediatric heart surgery in "blue babies.")

In 1965, Japanese doctors used HBOT to treat carbon monoxide poisoning from a coal mine fire. The oxygen displaced the carbon monoxide in the red blood cells. Scientists also found that burns healed faster when patients were treated with HBOT, generating yet another use for the therapy. We now know that oxygen can reduce the secondary inflammation that accompanies any injury by activating the immune system's white blood cells and their discharge of toxic chemicals and enzymes, which further damages tissue.

Hyperbaric medicine finally gained full recognition by physicians for treating the bends. Dan Greathouse's story about his decompression sickness (see chapter 7), illustrates how HBOT can save the lives of divers. Diving medicine is the one area where there is universal acceptance of hyperbaric treatment, and it remains the go-to treatment for both recreational and occupational scuba divers.

What Are the FDA-Approved Uses for HBOT?

The Undersea and Hyperbaric Medical Society, an organization that represents physicians, nurses, and clinicians in the field of hyperbaric medicine, met with the Food and Drug

Administration (FDA) in the '70s and recommended HBOT for 13 conditions. Unfortunately, more than 40 years later, only one new indication has been added to this list (see below) despite the fact that HBOT has been shown to work for many others.

Keep in mind that just because the FDA has recognized only 14 indications to date, this doesn't mean that HBOT isn't being prescribed with great success for what is called "off label" use (conditions other than what is FDA approved). Take Botox, for example, which was originally developed to treat migraines and is now being widely used by dermatologists to erase wrinkles. Like countless new medications that are awaiting FDA approval, HBOT has stayed under the radar because the medical establishment often takes time to catch up with scientific innovation. To give you an idea of how behind the curve we are in the United States, hyperbaric therapy is approved for 73 conditions in Russia, where hundreds of studies have proven its efficacy. Other countries, including, China, Cuba, England, Asia, Israel, and South America, are also using hyperbaric therapy for diseases and conditions far beyond America's short list. The following is the current list of FDA-approved indications for HBOT that are covered by most insurance companies and Medicare:

1. **Air or gas embolism:** An air or gas embolism is caused by air in the arteries when diving or by an invasive medical procedure that punctures an artery or lung.
2. **Carbon monoxide poisoning:** Carbon monoxide (CO) poisoning or CO poisoning complicated by

cyanide poisoning. Also includes poisoning from meth-
ylene chloride.

3. **Gas gangrene:** The medical names for these severe
   infections of the muscle are clostridial myositis and
   myonecrosis.

4. **Crush injury:** Acute ischemias (loss of blood flow),
   typically caused by heavy equipment.

5. **Decompression sickness:** Decompression sickness is
   brought on when a diver ascends too quickly and does
   not allow the oxygen in the body to expand at a safe rate.

6. **Arterial insufficiencies:** This category includes
   wounds such as diabetic foot ulcers, which afflict one
   out of five people with type 2 diabetes and can lead to
   amputation. Recently added to this category was central retinal artery occlusion, or "stroke of the eye,"
   from blockages in the arteries of the eye.

7. **Severe anemia:** Severe anemia is any acute, major
   blood loss, including wounds on the battlefield or other
   traumas.

8. **Intracranial abscess:** Intracranial abscess is caused by
   an accumulation of infected material; these abscesses
   of the brain are common in patients with abnormal
   immune systems.

9. **Necrotizing soft tissue infections:** Caused by "flesh-
   eating bacteria," these severe infections usually progress rapidly.

10. **Osteomyelitis:** Chronic bone infections that resist
    standard treatment. Osteomyelitis occurs most often
    in the lower leg after severe trauma.

11. **Delayed radiation injury:** Radiation damages blood vessels, and the lack of blood supply can eventually cause wounds to form in the soft tissue and bones.

12. **Compromised skin grafts and flaps:** Grafts and flaps of skin and other tissue (cartilage, bone, fat) are used in reconstructive surgery (such as breast reconstruction after a mastectomy). In some cases, blood supply to the graft or flap is compromised, causing complications.

13. **Thermal burn injury:** Burns from fire or heat.

14. **Idiopathic sudden sensorineural hearing loss:** Classically defined as a hearing loss of at least 30 dB over at least three contiguous frequencies occurring within three days. This is the latest approved indication added by the Undersea and Hyperbaric Medical Society board of directors in 2011.

What Conditions/Illnesses Have You Used HBOT to Treat?

The chart on page 11 shows the indications for HBOT from internationally published reports and my own professional experience in the field.

What Does an HBOT Treatment Feel Like?

Think about how you feel when you are flying thousands of feet above the earth in an airplane. You might get a popping in your ears when there is a change in air pressure while inside the oxygen chamber. The HBOT patient lies still in the chamber for 60 to 90 minutes, the average length of time for a treatment.

Abstracts: 4th International Symposium on HBOT in
Cerebral Palsy and the Brain Injured Child
Ft. Lauderdale, Florida, July 25-30, 2004

Updated Table Presented THE AWAKENING
Hyperbaric Medical Symposium, San Jose, California, August 27, 2005

Revised for Hyperbaric Oxygen Therapy and the Recoverable Brain
8th International Symposium, July 23-28, 2008
The Importance of Hyperbaric Oxygen Therapy (HBOT) In Modern Medicine

William S. Maxfield, M.D., FACNM
8947 Donna Lu Drive, Odessa, Florida 33556
wsm@williamsmaxfieldmd.com

These indications for HBOT are obtained from the world literature and personal experience

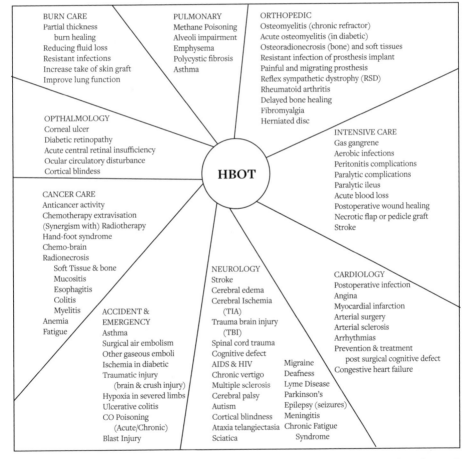

BURN CARE
Partial thickness
   burn healing
Reducing fluid loss
Resistant infections
Increase take of skin graft
Improve lung function

PULMONARY
Methane Poisoning
Alveoli impairment
Emphysema
Polycystic fibrosis
Asthma

ORTHOPEDIC
Osteomyelitis (chronic refractor)
Acute osteomyelitis (in diabetic)
Osteoradionecrosis (bone) and soft tissues
Resistant infection of prosthesis implant
Painful and migrating prosthesis
Reflex sympathetic dystrophy (RSD)
Rheumatoid arthritis
Delayed bone healing
Fibromyalgia
Herniated disc

OPTHALMOLOGY
Corneal ulcer
Diabetic retinopathy
Acute central retinal insufficiency
Ocular circulatory disturbance
Cortical blindess

INTENSIVE CARE
Gas gangrene
Aerobic infections
Peritonitis complications
Paralytic complications
Paralytic ileus
Acute blood loss
Postoperative wound healing
Necrotic flap or pedicle graft
Stroke

CANCER CARE
Anticancer activity
Chemotherapy extravasation
(Synergism with) Radiotherapy
Hand-foot syndrome
Chemo-brain
Radionecrosis
   Soft Tissue & bone
   Mucositis
   Esophagitis
   Colitis
   Myelitis
Anemia
Fatigue

HBOT

**ACCIDENT &
EMERGENCY**
Asthma
Surgical air embolism
Other gaseous emboli
Ischemia in diabetic
Traumatic injury
   (brain & crush injury)
Hypoxia in severed limbs
Ulcerative colitis
CO Poisoning
   (Acute/Chronic)
Blast Injury

NEUROLOGY
Stroke
Cerebral edema
Cerebral Ischemia
   (TIA)
Trauma brain injury
   (TBI)
Spinal cord trauma
Cognitive defect
AIDS & HIV
Chronic vertigo
Multiple sclerosis
Cerebral palsy
Autism
Cortical blindness
Ataxia telangiectasia
Sciatica

Migraine
Deafness
Lyme Disease
Parkinson's
Epilepsy (seizures)
Meningitis
Chronic Fatigue
   Syndrome

CARDIOLOGY
Postoperative infection
Angina
Myocardial infarction
Arterial surgery
Arterial sclerosis
Arrhythmias
Prevention & treatment
   post surgical cognitive defect
Congestive heart failure

NOTE: Stem cell therapy may impact all segments of medical care. There is every reason to believe HBOT as supportive therapy for stem cell treatment will be as beneficial as HBOT has been in improving the results of skin and pedicle grafts, especially since data now shows that HBOT increases the stem cell population of the body by a factor of eight.

How Often Is HBOT Given?

The number of treatments depends on the individual case and rate of recovery. Most treatments are given once a day, five days a week. Some people have treatments twice a day.

Are There Potential Side Effects or Contraindications with HBOT?

There are a few side effects and contraindications with HBOT and most are minor. I recommend, however, that patients with emphysema get chest X-rays prior to treatment to check for what's called an "emphysematous bleb." Emphysema is difficulty breathing due to air trapped in the lung, resulting in reduced lung capacity. The lung contains many millions of tiny air sacs. As we breathe in, oxygen moves from the air sacs into the blood in the capillaries. If an air sac within the lung ruptures, air can escape into surrounding tissue, forming a bubble or scar tissue around the bleb. When this occurs, the bleb no longer has the ability to perform gas exchange.

There is also a 1 in 10,000 chance of a patient having a seizure, so this reaction is rare. If this happens, the air pressure is lowered to resolve the seizure. If you are being treated for seizures, you might have an increased risk of having a seizure during treatment.

Some patients notice a slight change in vision after HBOT due to the pressure in the eyes, but many have reported improved vision, which I discuss later in the book. Claustrophobia is perhaps the most common problem for people who do not like being in an enclosed oxygen chamber. For these people, sedatives can help them relax during the procedure. Nearly everyone becomes accustomed to the chamber with time, and most side effects go away after the treatment is over.[2]

What Are the Different Types of Oxygen Chambers?

There are monoplace oxygen chambers as well as soft-side, hard-side, and multiplace chambers. Monoplace chambers are designed to treat one person pressurized with 100 percent oxygen. Multiplace chambers are designed to hold several people at a time (there's one that seats up to 12 people), and oxygen is delivered through a mask or a hood. All chambers are clear-sided so you can watch TV and allow for two-way communication with the technician.

Hard-side chambers are made of acrylic, and soft-sided chambers are inflatable, but they do not provide the same benefits as hard chambers. HBOT given in a hard chamber can regrow bone and tissue in severely damaged areas of the body. They are made to go to pressures that heal. Soft-sided chambers were first designed to temporarily treat divers and mountain climbers en route to a hard chamber. Treatment provided in a hard chamber is supported by thousands of clinical studies, and it is the method recognized for reimbursement by insurance companies and the federal government.

Do not bring anything that will cause a spark or fire into an oxygen chamber, such as watches, belt buckles, jewelry, batteries, metals, or cell phones. Patients should always wear all-cotton materials and no polyester or synthetic fibers. My patients usually wear surgical scrubs. Some people wear hospital gowns. People whose symptoms can be controlled at pressures of 1.25 to 1.3 ATA can buy and use a chamber at home.

What Is the Cost of HBOT?

It is more expensive to get HBOT in a hospital chamber ($2,000 an hour) than it is in an outpatient clinic ($200 an hour), but depending on the condition, it might be better to be in a hospital setting. Because most dives last approximately two hours from beginning to end, and most patients need multiple treatments (an average of 20, not counting follow-up maintenance), you should do the math to determine which option is best. Given the expense hyperbaric treatments, clinics might be preferable if your condition does not require in-patient care and is not covered by insurance.

One of my patients was a veteran who lost a leg in an improvised explosive device (IED) blast. His other leg was badly damaged and in jeopardy of being amputated. A leg amputation costs approximately $90,000, plus the price of the prosthesis. He opted for 23 HBOT treatments in a hospital instead of amputation, which came to $23,000, a significant savings, and, more important, ultimately saved his remaining leg, which his doctors thought he would lose. He is now able to walk on his wounded leg. In spite of stories like this one, many veteran hospitals are cutting back on hyperbaric therapy for reasons that are difficult to fathom.

Will Insurance and Medicare Pay for HBOT Treatments?

The FDA-approved conditions will be at least partly covered by most insurance providers, but check with your insurance company to see if your condition is eligible. Some patients have appealed and won coverage when submitting proof of efficacy. People with Medicare Part B will get 80 percent of HBOT treatments covered for the following with some provisos, including that the procedure must be administered in a single-person oxygen chamber:

- acute carbon monoxide intoxication
- decompression illness
- gas embolism
- gas gangrene
- acute traumatic peripheral ischemia
- crush injuries and suturing of severed limbs
- progressive necrotizing infections
- acute peripheral arterial insufficiency
- preparation and preservation of compromised skin grafts
- chronic refractory osteomyelitis, unresponsive to conventional medical and surgical management
- osteoradionecrosis as an adjunct to conventional treatment
- soft tissue radionecrosis as an adjunct to conventional treatment
- cyanide poisoning
- actinomycosis, a long-term infection that causes sores or abscesses in the body's soft tissues, including the

mouth, nose, and throat (HBOT is covered only as an adjunct to conventional therapy when the disease process is resistant to antibiotics and surgical treatment.)

- diabetic wounds of the lower extremities if you meet these three criteria:
  1. You have type 1 or type 2 diabetes and have a lower extremity wound that's due to diabetes.
  2. You have a wound classified as Wagner grade III or higher.
  3. You've failed an adequate course of standard wound therapy.

If you get nonemergency HBOT from a facility in Illinois, Michigan, or New Jersey, you may need to get prior authorization for Medicare to cover your HBOT services. You or your facility may send a request for prior authorization to Medicare before you get these services. To do this, you must submit medical records to show that the HBOT is medically necessary. For more information on coverage, call 1-800-MEDICARE.[3]

What Are the Biggest Misconceptions about HBOT?

The biggest misconception is that hyperbaric oxygen therapy is not science. The second myth is that it doesn't work, and the third is that it's quackery. The truth is that HBOT is based on hard science, and it is a therapy for wounds in any location and for any duration.

Why and How Are Scans Used as Part of the HBOT Treatment?

Brain and body imaging is an important part of HBOT because it allows doctors to determine how much damage the patient has when he or she walks into the office, as well as to see and quantify the effects of the treatments. By looking at scans, we can also decide how many treatments are needed. You can submit the before-and-after scans and other records to your insurance provider as evidence that the therapy works. The following are some of the most common medical scans used:

SPECT: A single-photon emission computerized tomography (SPECT) scan uses a radioactive substance and a special camera to look at blood flow and activity in the brain as 3-D maps. This type of scan is used most often by HBOT practitioners, especially when treating traumatic brain injuries. A SPECT scan tells us three things: good activity, too little activity, or too much activity. SPECT imaging has been indispensable for proving the efficacy of HBOT because it can clearly illustrate a marked difference in brain activity before and after HBOT treatments. Some traditional doctors do not accept SPECT scan results due to resolution quality, but in numerous cases that I and other HBOT practitioners have seen show marked improvement in cognitive brain function using SPECT scans.

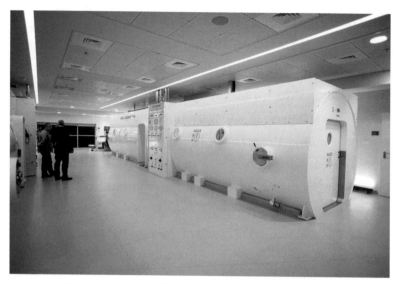

Source: Dr. Maxfield and Mayo Clinic

MRIs: A magnetic resonance imaging (MRI) scan is an imaging test that uses powerful magnets and radio waves to
take pictures of organs and structures inside the brain and
body. MRI scans are useful for examining the brain and spinal cord, and they are used to diagnose a variety of conditions, from torn ligaments to tumors. Single MRI images
are called slices. The images can be stored on a computer
or printed on film. One exam produces dozens or sometimes hundreds of images.

A functional MRI (fMRI) is a neuroimaging procedure that uses MRI technology to measure brain activity
by detecting changes associated with blood flow. Some
MRI machines make a lot of noise, so ask the radiologist
for earplugs if you are bothered by this. During the scan,
which is painless, you must lie still on a table that slides

inside a tunnel-shaped machine. Some people feel claustrophobic in closed MRIs. If this is the case for you, look for a facility that has an open machine or use a sedative before the procedure to help calm you down. Before you get a scan, tell your doctor if any of the following apply to you:

- You are pregnant.
- You have pieces of metal in your body, such as shrapnel, a bullet injury, or from work-related injuries.
- You have metal or electronic devices in your body, such as a cardiac pacemaker or a metal artificial joint.[4]

CT: A computerized tomography (CT or CAT) scan combines a series of X-ray images taken from different angles and uses computer processing to examine blood vessels and soft tissues inside the body and brain. CT scans allow the doctor to look at the inside of the body just as one would look at the inside of a loaf of bread by slicing it. This type of special X-ray, in a sense, takes "pictures" of slices of the body so doctors can examine the area of interest.

CT scans are frequently used to evaluate the brain, neck, spine, chest, abdomen, pelvis, and sinuses. It is especially useful when examining internal injuries from car accidents or other types of trauma. A CT scan can be used to visualize nearly all parts of the body and to diagnose a disease or injury or plan medical, surgical, or radiation treatments.[5]

PET: A positron emission tomography (PET) scan helps reveal how your tissues and organs are functioning. A radioactive drug called a "tracer" may be injected, swallowed, or inhaled, depending on which organ or tissue is being examined. The tracer collects in areas of your body that have higher levels of chemical activity, which often correspond to areas of disease. These areas show up as bright spots on a PET scan. It is useful in testing for some cancers, heart disease, and brain disorders.[6]

Is HBOT Taught in Medical Schools, and Why Is the Medical Establishment Reluctant to Recognize the Significance of HBOT?

Four years ago, Dr. Harch and one of his colleagues did a survey of 75 medical schools to see how many include hyperbaric medicine as part of their curriculum. Much to their dismay, three quarters of the respondents did not teach hyperbaric medicine. The other 25 percent offered a workshop or lecture. That's it. When I went to medical school in the '50s, we were told that HBOT was voodoo medicine and charlatanism. My generation of doctors (i.e., old-school) did not have the proper education about HBOT and, to this day, many physicians are stubbornly opposed to using it even as a complementary treatment. Things are beginning to improve within medical education, but there's a long way to go in terms of teaching doctors about HBOT. Until then, as I said in the beginning of this book, HBOT needs to be driven by patient demand because there is still a perception problem when it comes to hyperbaric oxygen therapy.

Another reason HBOT has been kept under wraps, especially in this country, is economic. Many surgeons and hospitals where procedures are performed are reluctant to promote HBOT because nonmedicinal and noninvasive options will reduce the need for medications and surgery, which cuts into hospital, university, and health care provider profits. The medical establishment continues to stall by demanding more clinical studies, and it refuses to accept studies that prove HBOT works. Even when medical research shows that HBOT should be the preferred method of treatment, it is not done. Clinical studies are expensive, and there is not enough funding for hyperbaric medicine if you don't have the deep pockets of a for-profit industry like Big Pharma, which pays for much of the research and development at universities and hospitals.

It is probably not a coincidence that many of the countries that do the most HBOT treatments are those that also have some form of socialized medicine. The Moscow Hyperbaric Center, for example, has about 80 oxygen chambers.

"Much of the rejection of hyperbaric oxygen therapy is rooted in fear," said Dr. Philip James, professor of hyperbaric medicine at the University of Dundee, Scotland, when interviewed by a reporter for the *Telegraph* in 2015. "Fear of the physics involved, the equipment, even fear of entering a pressure chamber." Dr. James, one of the United Kingdom's foremost hyperbaric oxygen experts and author of *Oxygen and the Brain*, has spent most of his professional life involved in deep-sea diving, where high levels of oxygen are routinely used for brain and spinal cord injuries. "Until oxygen therapy is taught in our medical schools, doctors will continue to be uninformed of the critical importance of oxygen in healing," he continued. "[HBOT] has not made headlines, but it ranks alongside the discovery of the structure of DNA and is set to define a new era in the treatment of injury and disease."[7]

Have There Been Scientific Studies Verifying the Effectiveness of HBOT?

There have been hundreds of studies on HBOT conducted around the world that prove it works, and I've included just a few of them at the end of this book. In 1981, Russia presented more than 300 studies with hundreds of patients at the Seventh Annual Hyperbaric Conference. Equine studies currently being done in Russia also found HBOT to be a viable treatment for a type of pneumonia that both horses and human share. Hundreds more new studies have been done since then, including many from China.

In 2016, Thomas Fox, a member of the American Association of Hyperbaric Awareness task force and a certified hyperbaric oxygen practitioner based in Montreal, Canada, presented a number of studies on the use of HBOT for war-related injuries to the Department of Defense. He intends to continue meeting with the Department of Defense until hyperbaric oxygen therapy is fully embraced by the Veterans

Administration. (See chapter 7 for Tom's story about his stepsons with cerebral palsy and for the section "Healing Our Wounded Warriors.")

Some Basic Biology

Red Blood Cells

Not everyone understands the different types of cells that make up our body and bloodstream and the role they play in our health and healing. Here is a basic primer:

- Red blood cells are what give our blood that red color by carrying oxygen around the body. Think of them as a breath of fresh air for your body.
- They are a round cell with no nucleus, but they are full of iron.
- They use an iron-rich chemical called hemoglobin to pick up the oxygen from the lungs. When they are full of oxygen, they turn bright scarlet. When the blood is full of carbon-dioxide waste that is discarded by the cells, they appear much darker.
- Just one drop of blood contains 5 million red blood cells, so imagine how many there are in the 1.3 gallons (5 liters) coursing

through your body. They are produced in the marrow inside your bones, which pumps out 2 million red blood cells every second. When an aging red blood cell gets broken down, its red color will end up as the "yellow" in urine.

White Blood Cells (B Cell)

White blood cells are also known as B cells. The B cells protect you from future invasions that make you sick. They are like the body's police that patrol the blood and lymphatic systems looking for trouble. White blood cells

- highlight dangerous invaders with markers called antibodies
- release chemical flags that plant themselves on the invaders
- are markers that help destroy the invaders that make you sick
- are also called lymphocytes
- are called lymphoma when cancerous

T Cells

T cells are white blood cells that work in the immune system. Like the B cell, they are designed to kill invaders that make you sick. T cells

- stand for "thymus cells"
- do battle in the lymphatic system and in the blood, like natural-born killers
- cruise around your body's blood vessels looking for invaders such as bacteria and viruses, including the flu. When you get sick, there can be as many as 7,000 T cells in one drop of blood. The B cell guides the T cell to the right target
- can become diseased by HIV and attacked by the virus

Stem Cells

Stem cells are unlike any other cell—brain cells are always brain cells, and red blood cells can never become anything else—but stem cells can grow into any type of cell (kidney, heart, liver, or skin) or just keep reproducing. Because of their adaptability, stem cells might be used one day to build replacement organs. Transplants or grafts grown from stem cells in a lab are also possible. They can even be used to repair faulty DNA, which causes some of the scariest diseases such as Alzheimer's and Parkinson's. Stem cells

- can morph and grow into anything
- are found in embryos, bone marrow, the liver, and the eyes
- can someday be used to build replacement body parts

2

EMERGENCY/
WOUND CARE

· ·

Some of you might recall the 1987 news story about Jessica
McClure, a little girl who was trapped in a well and rescued
after two and a half days. She was rushed to a hospital in Texas
that happened to have a hyperbaric oxygen chamber. The doctors who evaluated her injuries thought she would lose her
entire right foot, but after HBOT treatments, she walked out
of the hospital having lost only the tip of her pinky toe.

The case created a swirl of controversy when a letter
appeared in the *Journal of the American Medical Association*
stating that HBOT was not the correct course of action for

injuries like Jessica's. This misguided conclusion ignored thousands of cases like Jessica's, as well an animal study released at the time that proved conclusively that hyperbaric oxygen is effective in wound healing. Unfortunately, the animal study was not publicized in the media, so the value of Jessica's hyperbaric oxygen treatment was never widely known or accepted by the medical community or the public.

A little known fact is that the only reason Jessica had access to HBOT after her accident was because of a private donor whose daughter had multiple sclerosis (MS). The girl's father was tired of commuting to Dallas for HBOT treatments, so he bought an oxygen chamber for their local hospital, which is where Jessica was also treated. As far as I know, this girl was the only patient with MS to be treated in this chamber. Tragically, when the father was later diagnosed with degenerative and fatal ALS (a.k.a. Lou Gehrig's disease), he was denied treatment in the very chamber he had donated to the hospital.

Hyperbaric oxygen therapy as a treatment for wounds has been woefully misunderstood for hundreds of years. "Hyperbaric oxygen therapy exerts its wound-healing effects by expression and suppression of thousands of genes," Dr. Paul Harch, the New Orleans–based HBOT specialist, explains. "It increases the anti-inflammatory genes and decreases the pro-inflammatory genes through oxygen pressure regulation." The genetic reaction triggered by HBOT is part of its miraculous healing powers.[1]

FACT: Hyperbaric oxygen is not only good for crush injuries like Jessica McClure's; it can help speed up the healing process for both minor and severe fractures.

Don't Get Burned: Burn Care

HBOT is often used for what is called "thermal" burn cases (commonly known as second- and third-degree burns). Thermal burns are caused by any external heat source, such as a flame from an open fireplace, a house fire, a scald from steam or hot liquid, or direct contact with a hot object such as an oven rack or stove. One of the most serious consequences is the threat of infection, which can lead to illness or even death. While traditional medicine often calls for the use of antibiotics when treating burns, they might not work against bacteria that have developed a resistance to drugs.

In third-degree burns, the initial injury is followed by tissue loss. This means that the surrounding tissue also becomes damaged because blood vessels have been destroyed. When this happens, downstream blood flow from the site is stopped, which creates further tissue death due to a lack of oxygen. At this point, the body does not recognize the tissue as its own and perceives it as a harmful invader. This jeopardized tissue becomes a target for the immune system, which "attacks" the dying and surrounding tissues, resulting in even more tissue death.

HBOT should be given within the first 48 to 72 hours to prevent the tissue damage from spreading beyond the initial area. By supplying the body with added oxygen—up to

12 times that of breathing air at sea level—the damaged area can be brought "back to life." Hyperbaric oxygen signals to the body that the tissue is no longer a foreign invader, allowing the normal wound-healing processes to take place.

But HBOT treatments for burns shouldn't stop there. Beyond 72 hours, HBOT helps by continuing to promote new tissue growth, which encourages healing by helping manufacture new blood vessels, which, in turn, is responsible for collagen production. In addition, HBOT reduces the body's inflammation that would otherwise slow down the healing process. Finally, HBOT offers infection control, as oxygen is the white blood cells' weapon against bacteria.

When used in addition to traditional treatments, hyperbaric oxygen therapy can slow the progression of skin and lung damage and reduce swelling. HBOT is considered safe even for patients with severe and extensive burns. By helping the body fight infection, hyperbaric oxygen can improve healing, lessen damage from infection, and thereby decrease the chances of death in severe cases. It can also reduce healing time and lessen scarring.

If you are undergoing skin grafts, consider immediate HBOT to help with the healing process. Skin grafts tend to be unsuccessful when the body has insufficient oxygen, and an abundance of oxygen has been shown to increase success for skin grafts.

The benefits of HBOT for burn victims cannot be understated. Because not all physicians are knowledgeable about HBOT, tell your doctor or emergency medical services team to take you to a hospital that has a hyperbaric oxygen chamber immediately! Emergency doctors are usually familiar with HBOT but, if not, demand, don't ask. The sooner you get treatment, the better your outcome.

Degrees of Burns

- **First degree:** A first-degree, or superficial, burn affects only the epidermis (top layer of the skin). The burn site is red, painful, and dry with no blistering. A mild sunburn or match burn are examples of first-degree burns. Long-term tissue damage is rare and usually consists of a lightening or a darkening in the skin color.
- **Second degree:** With a second-degree, or partial-thickness, burn, the epidermis and part of the dermis (lower layer of the skin) are both damaged. The burn site appears red and blistered and may be swollen and painful.
- **Third degree:** With a third-degree, or full-thickness, burn, the epidermis and dermis are destroyed. Burns where there is also damage to the underlying tendon, muscle, and bone are considered to be third degree.
- **Fourth degree:** With a fourth-degree burn, the burn site appears white or charred and

no sensation is felt in the area because the nerve endings and the blood vessels carrying needed oxygen have been destroyed. Unlike third-degree burns, fourth-degree burns can damage the tendons, muscles, and bones.

Approved Indications for Wound Treatment with HBOT

Gas gangrene: This condition results from dirty wounds inflicted in battle or punctures from rusty metal. It is a rapidly progressive infection of the muscle that is life-threatening unless treated with antibiotics, aggressive surgery, amputation, or HBOT.

Crush injuries: These injuries are usually caused by heavy equipment falling onto the extremities, resulting in crushing and loss of blood flow. With swelling from the crush, blood flow is further compromised and the muscle compartments become gangrenous.

Anaerobic infections: Anaerobic bacteria can infect the tissues in deep wounds and internal organs where there is little oxygen. These infections are characterized by abscess formation, foul-smelling pus, and tissue destruction.

If You Need Intensive Care

According to a 2011 article that appeared in *Critical Care Medicine*, data from research and clinical trials on the use of hyperbaric medicine when treating critically ill patients showed that hyperbaric oxygen can be helpful for a number of intensive care conditions, including gas gangrene and acute crush injuries. The report went on to note that most hospitals are not equipped with oxygen chambers or doctors who are properly trained in HBOT. If this is the case, intensive care patients in need of hyperbaric oxygen treatments should go to clinics operated by specialists in HBOT.

The report concluded that, as in all medical interventions, it is important to consider the risk versus benefit of hyperbaric oxygen for any given critical care disorder, but hyperbaric oxygen can be delivered safely to critically ill patients. Hospitals currently without hyperbaric oxygen capability should consider adding oxygen chambers to its facilities in order to treat patients for approved indications.

Diabetic Foot Ulcers

A diabetic ulcer is an open sore or wound that occurs in approximately 15 percent of patients with diabetes and is commonly located on the bottom of the foot. Of those who develop a foot ulcer, 6 percent will be hospitalized due to infection or other related complications. Diabetic foot ulcers are the most common reason for hospital stays for people with diabetes.

Hyperbaric oxygen therapy was found to be an effective treatment for "problem wounds" such as diabetic foot ulcers, according to the first controlled trial for this indication reported in *Diabetes Care* more than 20 years ago. The study found that HBOT's beneficial effects include a reduced risk of amputation in diabetic patients with foot wounds and an increased likelihood of wound healing.

Another randomized study published in 2008 compared the effects of HBOT with standard wound care alone on 100 patients with a diabetic foot ulcer that had not responded to a month of appropriate treatment. Researchers found that HBOT produced significantly higher rates of wound healing and lower rates of surgical interventions (amputations, skin flaps, or grafts).

Based on these published studies and my own professional experience, it is clear that HBOT improves long-term healing for chronic diabetic foot wounds that do not respond to other traditional therapy.[2]

Bone Infections

Osteomyelitis is the technical term for a bone infection that can travel through the bloodstream and spread from nearby tissue. Infections can also begin in the bone itself if an injury causes it to become exposed to germs. In children, osteomyelitis most commonly affects the bones of the legs and upper arms. In adults, it can infect the spine or vertebrae. Diabetics can develop osteomyelitis in their feet if they have foot ulcers. Once considered incurable, the traditional course of treatment is surgery to remove parts of the bone that have died, along with a strong course of antibiotics, often delivered intravenously and typically lasting from four to six weeks.

The good news for those with bone infections, including diabetic foot ulcers, is that HBOT is not only an effective treatment but also FDA approved. It is especially useful when the immune system is not functioning properly. I've used HBOT in my practice for diabetic patients, one of whom was referred to me by an orthopedic surgeon after developing an infection in his foot. The problem was so severe that his doctor considered amputation. After coming to me for HBOT treatments, I was able to save this man's foot. (Interestingly, despite the success of my treatment, I never got another recommendation from this patient's orthopedic surgeon again.)

I had another patient who was a young soldier scheduled to have his leg amputated after having developed an infection. After 25 HBOT treatments, we were able to save his leg. I have also found HBOT can help patients with a prosthesis that has become too painful to bear. Sometimes the prosthesis causes a bone fracture when it rubs around at the tip, and HBOT creates a level of cortical bone that prevents this friction from happening.

Reducing Wound Pain

Wounds can hurt—a lot—but the amount of pain depends on the type of the injury, its location, and the severity. Burns are particularly painful, of course. Although a cut, scrape, or puncture wound may hurt less, it can become serious if left untreated. Whatever kind of wound, you should follow these steps:

- Take care of the injury immediately because even a minor wound can get infected if bacteria are allowed to build up in the injured site. If the wound is minor, you can apply first aid, such as antibacterial ointment or cream at home.

- If you get a puncture wound or step on a rusty nail, you must see a doctor immediately because you may need a tetanus shot. Most people are not up-to-date on their tetanus vaccines, if they've had them at all, so don't take chances by trying to tough it out. Call your doctor or go to a local urgent care center. The same goes for puncture wounds from an animal bite—seek emergency medical attention. If you have a deep cut or one with jagged edges, stitches may be needed to close the wound.

- Clean the wound with water. Avoid using soap, hydrogen peroxide, or iodine, which can irritate the injury. Hold the wound under running water to remove dirt, and use sterilized tweezers (boil them first) to remove any remaining debris. If you can't clean the wound yourself, see a doctor, because the dirt could trigger an infection. If there is a large object embedded in the wound, don't try to remove it—seek emergency medical attention.

- After the wound is clean, apply antibiotic ointment one to three times a day to prevent infection, and cover it with a sterile bandage. Before reapplying ointment, clean the wound. Stop using the ointment if you develop a rash or other reaction and call your doctor. Change the bandage daily, and use soap to clean the skin *around* the wound.

- If the injury doesn't stop bleeding on its own, use a clean cloth to apply pressure. Maintain the pressure for 20 minutes while elevating the wounded area. If bleeding continues after 20 minutes of pressure or blood spurts out of the wound, get medical help.

- Keep a close watch on the wound to make sure it's healing properly. If the wound does not begin to heal, feels warm, becomes inflamed, or the skin around it shows red streaks, seek immediate medical attention.[3]

3
HBOT AND AGING

· ·

One of the most exciting benefits of HBOT is the way it helps with conditions associated with aging, including dementia, eye problems, arthritis, and even, some say, thinning or wrinkled skin. Two renowned HBOT specialists, Dr. Richard Neubauer and Dr. Pavel Yutsis, collaborated on an article about their work in restoring brain function for people with dementia. They used SPECT scans to document the neurological changes after hyperbaric oxygen therapy.

In their article "New Frontiers: Anti-Aging Properties of Hyperbaric Oxygen Therapy," published in July 2009 by

Townsend Letter for Doctors and Patients, Dr. Neubauer explained how HBOT helps reactivate the part of the brain that has been damaged by diminishing oxygen supply so that vascular dementia can be alleviated, and even eliminated. They described several patients, whom they treated for dementia, including the cases below.

D. L.'s Story

"D. L., a 70-year-old female, began to notice periods of confusion, forgetfulness, and agitation and had reached the point where she was unable to drive her car or live alone. Under most circumstances, a patient like this would be institutionalized in a care facility. Her daughter took her in. Both women were ministers in the Unity Church, but D. L. had lost her ability to work with parishioners.

A SPECT scan showed that D. L. did not have Alzheimer's disease but had hypoperfusion [decreased flow of oxygen] in the frontal and temporal lobes. She was given three treatments of hyperbaric oxygen and the scan was repeated. The changes in perfusion were striking, and it paralleled her clinical progress. She then received a total of 33 treatments. After 20 treatments, the patient returned to a perfectly normal lifestyle; she was able to drive her car and return to the pulpit. A SPECT scan conducted upon completion of the treatments showed that the improvements remained intact. Two and a half years later, the patient was doing extremely well and has had three mainte-nance hyperbaric oxygen treatments."

J. D.'s Story

"A 79-year-old male, J. D., complained of dizziness all day for two and a half months. He had suffered a stroke a month previously and was hospitalized for three to four days with no therapy given. He reported problems with memory as well as pain and stiffness in the neck. A baseline SPECT scan showed multiple areas of hypometabolism [an abnormally low meta-bolic rate that causes the body to become sluggish] with the main deficit seen in the left temporal, occip-ital zone. After 10 hyperbaric treatments (one hour in duration), the patient reported that his memory was much improved, his pain was relieved, and he felt much stronger with increased energy. SPECT scans after 10 treatments showed significant improvement in the localization in the left frontal and both parietal regions. The uptake pattern was also less patchy in other areas."

D. F.'s Story

"D. F. was a bright and alert 72-year-old female who worked as a secretary for Dr. Neubauer. After becom-ing slightly dizzy and confused, she had a left carotid endarterectomy [a procedure to treat carotid artery disease; this disease occurs when fatty, waxy deposits build up in one of the carotid arteries]. She appeared to be fine after the operation and continued working for a time before retiring.

After a number of months passed, we received a phone call from her daughter, who said her mother was so confused, disoriented, dizzy, and weak that she [the daughter] was selling her apartment and moving in to take care of her. Because of this change, we had D. F. come in for SPECT scan. Subsequently she had four hyperbaric oxygen treatments (one hour in duration), followed by a repeat SPECT scan.

The results were dramatic. All the symptoms, including confusion and dizziness were gone, and D. F. was able to live alone once again. She continued to drive her car and take care of all personal affairs. Eighteen months later, she remained clinically stable."

As the above cases clearly show, the use of hyperbaric oxygen therapy has given people suffering from dementia a better quality of life. Their SPECT scans before and after HBOT documented and proved the changes that occurred in their brains.

"Restoring brain functioning is one of many important goals of anti-aging therapies," writes Dr. Neubauer, who first suggested in the late '70s that hyperbaric oxygen can reactivate the zone around a special region surrounding the central area of a stroke or brain injury site, known as the "ischemic penumbra." The diminished oxygen supply to the penumbra is one of a few causes for the loss or failure of bodily functions. Hyperbaric oxygen therapy may restore function in areas of the brain that are hypoxic (low in oxygen pressure) and are primarily vascular in origin. HBOT can be helpful even in cases that occurred 12 to 13 years before receiving treatment.

Aging and DNA

In his book *The Oxygen Revolution*, Dr. Paul Harch describes a patient in his early 70s who came to him with full-blown dementia. He explains why HBOT helped this man who had no family history of dementia.

"It's important to understand that normal aging is a DNA phenomenon and an accumulation of insults throughout our lifetime," Dr. Harch explains. "This patient smoked cigarettes and drank alcohol for years, and all these insults built up to the point where he couldn't function anymore. What he was suffering from was carbon dioxide poisoning. His lifestyle was essentially creating wounding insults to his brain and body. This is why making healthy lifestyle choices are a crucial factor in fighting ravages of age." (See the box "Lifestyle changes for a Healthier Mind and Body" on page 46.)

Still, nearly anyone—including those who do not smoke or abuse alcohol and drugs—who is fortunate enough to achieve senior citizenship status worries about the onset of dementia. Will it happen to me, they wonder, and, if so, when? Is it inevitable, and is there anything that can be done to slow down or reverse the damage? When we can't remember where we put our keys and parked our car, or when the name of an old friend sticks like a glue trap to the tip of our tongue, we fear that these are symptoms of impending dementia.

Let's start by defining what dementia is and how it differs from its nasty cousin, Alzheimer's disease. Dementia is an umbrella term for the loss of cognitive function, such as reasoning or memory, that is severe enough to interfere with daily life. There are different types of dementia, including Alzheimer's, which is a neurodegenerative disease that occurs when brain cells die off over time. Unfortunately, there is no cure for the disease at the moment.

The clinical definition of dementia is the loss of about 50 grams of brain tissue (the average human brain has between 1,100 and 1,300 grams of brain tissue, men having about 200 more grams than women). Dementia can also be caused by a series of strokes, alcohol and drug abuse, or head trauma (either a single injury or multiple blows), as well as infections such as AIDS.

According to 2016 statistics from the Alzheimer's Association, more than 5 million Americans are living with Alzheimer's and one in three seniors die with the disease or another form of dementia. The good news is that there have been cases where HBOT has helped those who are not yet in the advanced stages of dementia. If too much cognitive function has been lost and the patient is already completely disoriented or unresponsive, it is difficult to reverse the damage. But there have been reports of some extraordinary cases where there has been some improvement after a number of HBOT treatments.[1]

SPECT scans can often predict the results of HBOT in patients with dementia. According to clinical stats compiled by Dr. Harch, if a scan shows some improvement after only one HBOT treatment, there is roughly a 90 percent chance that the patient will improve with repeated HBOT treatments. If the scan is worse or shows no change, there is roughly a 50 percent chance that patients will improve, while the other half will show no change after 40 HBOT treatments.[2]

Could Oxygen Therapy Have Saved Robin Williams?

After the tragic death by suicide of beloved actor/comedian Robin Williams in 2014, an autopsy revealed that he suffered from Lewy body dementia (LBD), a progressive disorder that leads to a decline in thinking, reasoning, and independent function. The disease, which affects an estimated 1.4 million Americans, is caused by protein deposits called Lewy bodies in brain cells that govern thinking, memory, and motor control.

Symptoms of LBD include visual hallucinations, movement disorders, insomnia, and depression. Because LBD is difficult to detect and differentiate from other disorders, it often goes undiagnosed. Robin Williams's wife said the actor did not know he had LBD prior to his death.

I have seen hyperbaric oxygen therapy help control the symptoms of LBD, so I believe HBOT would probably have benefitted Williams. He could have undergone a SPECT scan to detect irregularities and areas of damage in his brain. When we look at these scans, we can determine that the problem is physical, not psychological. Like veterans with blast injuries, which I will discuss later, LBD patients often attempt suicide prior to treatment.

Had Robin Williams been correctly diagnosed, I believe that a HBOT course could have repaired his damaged brain cells (along with getting clean and sober, addiction being another problem Williams suffered from) and would have allowed him to return to a healthy, normal life.[3]

Dealing with Dementia

The following are some helpful homespun tips for caregivers of those with dementia that have been circulating on the Internet and are of unknown origin. Many we know who are in this position have found this advice to be both helpful and comforting:

- Never argue; instead, agree.
- Never reason; instead, divert.
- Never lecture; instead, reassure.
- Never shame; instead, distract.
- Never say "remember"; instead, reminisce.
- Never say, "I told you"; instead, repeat/regroup.
- Never demand/command; instead, ask/model.
- Never say, "You can't"; say, "Do what you can."
- Never condescend; instead, encourage.
- Never force; instead, reinforce.

Lifestyle Changes for a Healthier Mind and Body

Nearly all doctors agree that you can reduce the risk of developing dementia by making some simple changes in your lifestyle. A review of 323 studies on Alzheimer's disease by researchers at the Memory and Aging Center at the University of California, San Francisco, gave the following seven lifestyle guidelines:

1. **Watch your waistline.** Ever notice how some people can have big bellies but lean legs or how women tend to store most of their fat in their thighs, hips, and butt? These are examples of fat distribution, which refers to where your body typically stores the fat, no matter what your weight is. This is important to note because where you store fat can be a predictor of health risk.

    If you have a high waist-to-hip ratio, for example, you are at greater risk of having late-onset Alzheimer's disease, according to a 2012 study of aging by the National Institutes of Health of 1,459 people ages 65 and up. The reason for this is fat that surrounds vital abdominal organs contributes to insulin resistance, lipid imbalances such as high triglycerides and low "good" high-density (HDL) cholesterol, and inflammation. Look in a full-length mirror to see where your fat is stored and if you are an apple, pear, or other shape.

2. **Keep your brain active.** As we age, it is easy to fall into a rut and do the same things day after day. But routines are not good for your brain or your memory. When our brain slips into autopilot, instead of forging new connections, we use the same neural pathways over and over again, like running on a hamster wheel. Our brains crave novelty, so mix it up a bit by having new experiences or learning something new, especially something that you enjoy doing.

    Many studies suggest that the more we are engaged in stimulating activities, the less likely we are to develop dementia. Eating at a different restaurant, learning a language or how to play an instrument, or even shopping at a different store or trying new kinds of food can keep your brain young and active. While crossword puzzles, Sudoku, and other brain-teasing games are thought to improve our mental acuity, solitary activities like these are not as good as those where we interact with other people. Start a bridge club in your area if there isn't one already, or join a neighborhood walking group.

3. **Lower your stress.** It is no surprise that chronic stress is bad for your health (both mental and physical). Cortisol, the so-called stress hormone, has been shown in animal studies to actually kill off neurons in the hippocampus, the brain's memory center. A study from the Rush Alzheimer's Disease Center in Chicago showed that people prone to stress were 2.4 times more likely to develop Alzheimer's disease than people who were not. Many other studies support the fact that those who suffer from anxiety and depression also have an increased risk of Alzheimer's. Meditation or yoga has been scientifically proven to lower cortisol levels and reduce stress, and practicing these for only 20 minutes a day can make a huge difference in your life.

4. **Rein in high blood pressure.** Blood pressure is measured by two numbers: The top number (systolic pressure) is the highest pressure inside your arteries, measured at the moment when your heart contracts. The bottom number (diastolic pressure) is the lowest pressure in your arteries, measured while your heart is relaxing

in between beats. Your ideal blood pressure should be less than 120/80. This may vary, however, depending on your age and other medical conditions. Discuss what the best blood pressure is for you with your doctor.

5. **Stay active.** The idea that exercise is good for your health is a no-brainer. But it has been scientifically proven that physical activity, especially the kind that gets your heart pumping and the blood circulating, is also good for your mind. The increased blood flow physically alters the brain, bathing it in a cascade of growth factors that regenerates brain cells and creates stronger neural connections. To achieve healthy circulation, ask your doctor to check your homocysteine level (associated with heart attack, stroke, and blood clots) and be aware of any atherosclerosis (hardening of the arteries) in your vascular system. A high homocysteine level can be treated with vitamin B complex, B12, and B6.

6. **Avoid smoking.** We all know that smoking is a risk factor for heart disease, stroke, lung cancer, and a multitude of other conditions. But did you know that smoking has been linked to dementia and Alzheimer's disease? It decreases blood flow to the brain, and the tobacco toxins promote inflammation. Breaking the habit can be difficult, but quitting cigarettes (including vapes and e-cigs) is arguably the single most important action you must take if you are truly serious about keeping your body and mind younger and healthier.

7. **Avoid high blood sugar.** A fasting blood sugar in the range of 100 to 125 indicates prediabetes, while a level higher than 126 indicates full-blown diabetes. In most cases, proper diet and exercise can lower blood sugar levels to the normal range. Often, losing as little as 5 to 10 pounds and being more active can make a significant difference to your health as you age.

8. **Get more sleep.** When you don't get enough sleep, does your mind tend to wander? Do you feel foggy and forgetful? Most of us experience symptoms like these when we don't get enough Zzzzs, and it's nothing to worry about if this is an infrequent occurrence. But chronic sleep deprivation can cause serious medical problems, including high blood pressure, heart disease, diabetes, unhealthy cholesterol levels, a weakened immune system, increased risk of infections, and even dementia. In one study, chronic sleep loss increased plaque formation in the brains of mice, one of the hallmarks of Alzheimer's. The message is clear—getting enough regular, restorative sleep is essential for keeping your brain healthy as you age.[4]

HBOT as Fountain of Youth

Aside from helping reverse some of the symptoms of dementia, anecdotal evidence has found that hyperbaric oxygen therapy can actually slow down some of the physical effects of aging. Valerie Greene, a stroke survivor and awareness leader, recalls meeting a 95-year-old woman at an HBOT clinic where both women were going for treatments.

"I saw a woman coming out of an HBOT chamber who didn't look sick at all," Valerie recalled. "I asked her what she was there for and she said she comes for the antiaging benefits. No joke—she was 95 and she looked 60! If people knew about the cosmetic benefits of HBOT, they would be lining up for time in the chamber!"

Antiaging is a little-known benefit of hyperbaric oxygen therapy because most patients get HBOT for other conditions described in this book. But time and time again, I see users of hyperbaric oxygen therapy looking younger after emerging from the chamber. "It can make your hair grow thicker," Valerie added, "and your sex drive will be off the charts. If people understood what oxygen does, you would have to make reservations months in advance to get into a chamber."

I ♥ HBOT:
HEART AILMENTS

In 1995, a man underwent six hours of surgery after a cardiac arrest. For years he suffered from severe memory loss and depression. More than a decade after his operation, he was referred to me. Not surprisingly, SPECT scans revealed abnormal activity in the brain. After 40 HBOT treatments, his scans showed marked improvement in both brain hemispheres. His memory was restored and his depression disappeared.

Research has shown that nearly all patients undergoing heart surgery could benefit from hyperbaric oxygen therapy. Over the past 10 years, multiple studies have shown that a third of bypass patients have persistent neurological and cognitive problems. This is caused by air bubbles from the bypass machine that enter the arterial circulation. Scans actually reveal bubbles going to into the brain. As a result, patients can develop decompression sickness. In a 2005 British study published in the *Journal of Thoracic and Cardiovascular Surgery*, scientists found that patients given several hyperbaric treatments prior to bypass surgery had a significant reduction in cognitive problems and inflammatory blood markers when compared with patients not receiving the HBOT.

In this country, hyperbaric oxygen is used primarily to treat infections and nonhealing bone in the sternum after a cardiovascular operation. Outside the United States, however, HBOT has been used to treat angina, myocardial infarction, arrhythmias, and congestive heart failure. In Russia, many patients with cardiac conditions opt for hyperbaric oxygen over surgical transplants. The increased use of stem cells might account for the spike in HBOT treatments for transplants in other countries, while the United States is still playing catch up because the FDA has not approved stem cell use.

Fact: For patients receiving bypass surgery, just two HBOT treatments have been shown to result in a 61 percent reduction in complications and a 20 percent reduction in intensive care unit stays.[1]

Jackie Brenner's Story: Atrial Fibrillation (A-Fib)

"In 2006, I was diagnosed with atrial fibrillation, which is when the heart beats irregularly. I was 57 at the time.

My heart would race so quickly it would hit the 180- to 200-beats-per-minute range and just lay me out. These runs could last up to eight hours. It would wake me up at 4 a.m. or I'd feel like I was about to pass out. You could actually see my heart pounding in my chest. It was so bad I couldn't function.

With atrial fibrillation, there is a risk of stroke when the blood pools in the atrium and causes a clot. I live in New Orleans, and I was moving my father, who also had a-fib for years, into a nursing home after Katrina. That day my heart just went off. I immediately saw a specialist who said, 'Jackie, you are going to get worse in 10 years.'

I started doing research on how to treat my condition. Medications like antiarrhythmics don't work, and I wasn't a candidate for anticoagulants because I have a blood condition called hemophilia C [a mild form of hemophilia that prevents the blood from clotting]. I ended up going to the Cleveland Clinic, where researchers have been studying this condition. I asked for something that wouldn't just treat the symptoms but cure it. Surgery was also not an option. I discovered that there were triggers that set my heart off. Certain foods I am allergic to, such as kale, spinach, sweet potatoes, and vanilla, would put me in the hospital. The doctors also discovered that I had a hiatal hernia. Once I stopped eating those trigger foods and fixed my hernia, my a-fib subsided.

But during my research, I had come across HBOT studies done in Europe. I live in a city with one of the best HBOT doctors, Dr. Paul Harch, so I went to see him. He said he couldn't guarantee hyperbaric oxygen therapy would work, but he wanted to give it a try. He prescribed 40 treatments, and about three quarters of the way through, while I was in the oxygen chamber, I felt something in my chest. It was strong and it kind of scared me. I didn't go back into the chamber for about three days. But after that experience, my heart started to settle down and it suddenly began beating regularly.

I went back for the HBOT treatments and, more than 100 dives later, I am now a-fib-free! Of course, I was carefully monitored. If you overdo HBOT treatments, you can plateau and start to revert back to where you were in the beginning. Now I just go for boosters. Ten years out from my diagnosis, I'm without medication and I consider myself 100 percent cured. Every once in a while I get a momentary run, but it's usually triggered by something I've eaten. HBOT was the piece of the puzzle that allowed me to get better. Now I'm healthier than ever and life is good!"

What Is A-Fib?

Atrial fibrillation (A-tre-al fi-bri-LA-shun), or a-fib, is the most common type of arrhythmia (ah-RITH-me-ah), where the heart can beat too fast, too slow, or with an irregular rhythm. A-fib occurs if rapid, disorganized electrical signals cause the heart's two upper chambers—called the atria—to fibrillate. The term "fibrillate" means to contract fast and irregularly. In a-fib, blood pools in the atria if it isn't pumped properly into the heart's two lower chambers. As a result, the heart's upper and lower chambers don't work together as they should. People who have a-fib may not feel symptoms, but it can increase the risk of stroke. In some people, it can cause chest pain or heart failure, especially if the heart rhythm is extremely rapid.[2]

5
CANCER CARE

· ·

In the early '80s, a patient of mine named Marion, then 34 years old with two young children, was diagnosed with a sarcoma (a malignant tumor) the size of an egg located by her shoulder blade. Doctors gave her just five years to live. This is her story.

Marion Carter's Story: Sarcoma

"My doctor kept telling me the bump on my back was a fatty tumor and nothing to worry about. It concerned me, so I asked him to remove it anyway. As it turned out, it was a rare form of cancer, and I was given a

5 percent chance of living five more years. I'll never forget that phone call; I was so devastated. My doctor suggested I go to a special cancer facility in Houston. We knew about Dr. Maxfield because his brother was my father's physician. As a devout Christian, I felt that God led me to Dr. Maxfield and I would be fine.

Dr. Maxfield set me up with radiation treatments and gave me HBOT in his clinic before each radiation treatment. I also got hyperbaric oxygen *before* my surgery to help with the healing process. I had a wide excision that went all the way down to the bone and I needed a skin graft, which doctors warned me might not take at first. I believe that the HBOT helped because my skin graft took immediately. I still have a huge scar that makes people gasp if I wear a swimsuit, but I don't care because I'm alive today. After the surgery, I continued to get hyperbaric treatments and went back for maintenance every three months. A year after the operation, I was in 100 percent remission. Nearly 30 years later, I have still not had a reoccurrence of cancer.

I continued to return to the HBOT clinic in Florida for maintenance once a year, and now I'm finished. I'm 68 and I feel like I'm in my 40s. My husband and I are retired and living a wonderful life in Oklahoma. I wouldn't be here if it wasn't for Dr. Maxfield."

HBOT Cancer Studies

Although HBOT is by no means a cure for cancer, many clinical studies have shown hyperbaric oxygen therapy to be extremely effective with patients receiving cancer treatments. A 2010 Ohio State University study published in the *Journal of Cancer Biology and Therapy* found that hyperbaric oxygen could shrink ovarian tumors. Ninety-minute sessions for 21 days corrected the hypoxic tumor and apparently made chemo more effective.[1]

In an earlier study conducted in Norway, hyperbaric treatments alone were found to be twice as effective as chemotherapy in controlling breast cancer. One explanation for this is when oxygen-deprived cells are brought back to normal, cancer cells start dying out by apoptosis, which is the process of eliminating old, unnecessary, unhealthy cells without damaging the rest of the body. Aggressive chemotherapy can sometimes kill off the good cells as well as the bad.

Another study conducted at a Japanese university found a potential role for HBOT therapy in the treatment of malignant tumors and radiation injury of the brain. Nonrandomized clinical trials using chemotherapy combined with HBOT showed a significant increase in survival rates for patients with recurrent malignant gliomas. The possibilities of combining HBOT therapy with radiotherapy and/or chemotherapy to overcome newly diagnosed and recurrent malignant gliomas, researchers say, deserve more extensive clinical trials.

Scientists also say there is promising potential for the treatment and possibly prevention of radiation injury to the brain after radiosurgery for brain lesions using HBOT. The authors of a 2013 study wrote, "The possibilities with HBOT to enhance the therapeutic effect of irradiation and to even increase the radiation dose if there are ways to combat the side effects, should boost new scientific interest into the whole field of oncology looking for new medicines, equipment, and techniques available to medical practitioners in fighting cancer."[2]

Joe's Story: Postchemo Hand Syndrome

A patient of mine developed a swollen hand after receiving chemotherapy for lung cancer. The swelling was so severe that Joe couldn't bend his fingers, and his chemotherapist was concerned that he might lose the use of his entire hand. Joe, who was a carpenter, depended on his hands for his livelihood. He came to me for what he thought was a last resort. After just three HBOT treatments, the blood circulation in his hand increased to the point where he was able to bend his fingers again. The hyperbaric therapy along with a skin graft helped save his hand and his job.

Radiation Necrosis

Radiation necrosis is a postoperative condition in which a lesion forms at the site where a malignant tumor was originally removed. It can be a long-term central nervous system risk for patients who have undergone radiotherapy or radiosurgery. Fortunately, this is one of the approved conditions for HBOT in the United States, which is gaining acceptance among traditional physicians who once believed that hyperbaric oxygen would increase the growth of cancer cells, whereas the opposite is true. The fact is the use of HBOT has, in general, lowered the incidences of cancer recurrence, which has been documented in several animal studies.

A 2015 *Medscape* article by Dr. Michael J. Schneck, professor of neurology and neurosurgery at Loyola University, Chicago, says treating a patient with radiation necrosis with anticancer drugs is not the answer. In addition to observing and monitoring patients with a series of MRI scans, Dr. Schneck wrote, "For patients with signs and symptoms of mass effect, increased intracranial pressure, or neurologic disability, consider . . . surgical evaluation, steroids, anticoagulation, or hyperbaric oxygen therapy separately or in combination." Dr. Schneck also wrote that there are benefits of hyperbaric oxygen in treating this condition with 20 to 30 sessions for approximately 90 to 120 minutes with caveats, including the fact that HBOT is not readily available at many medical centers. He added, however, that some case studies found patients receiving steroid therapy along with HBOT "showed a resolution of a lesion on MRIs."[3]

There are also excellent data that show hyperbaric oxygen can decrease the effects of radiation and chemotherapy, including mucositis (a common side effect of chemotherapy and radiotherapy that involves the digestive tract) and colitis (inflammation of the inner lining of the colon) in patients in both acute and chronic stages. It is also beneficial for cancer patients whose tissues are damaged by radiation therapy, especially those who develop oxygen-deficient wounds that don't heal well. The reason for this is that hyperbaric oxygen promotes the release of growth hormones, which helps form blood vessels in irradiated tissue.

Chemo Brain

HBOT has been used successfully to treat other complications of cancer therapy such as "chemo brain," a common term used by cancer survivors to describe cognitive dysfunctions, such as fogginess and memory loss, caused by chemotherapy.

Olivia, a patient of mine who was diagnosed with breast cancer at the age of 64, spent six years after her chemotherapy and radiation treatments "living in a fog." Her short-term memory got progressively worse to the point where she could no longer work or perform even the most basic tasks at home. Studies confirm that 25 percent of breast cancer chemotherapy patients report mild to severe chemo brain.

Olivia's cognitive loss was so severe, however, that she was forced to go on disability. In 2002, she came to my office, where I gave her 20 HBOT treatments. Afterward, her memory returned and she was able to go back to work and resume her normal daily life. I have seen many patients like Olivia whose chemo brain was reduced or eliminated completely after HBOT treatments. If you are experiencing postchemo side effects, see if HBOT helps improve your cognitive function.

Consider Complementary Therapies

Although surgery, chemotherapy, and radiation are the traditional treatments for those with a cancer diagnosis, patients might want to consider a variety of "complementary" therapies that can help reduce their pain and anxiety during cancer care. Keep in mind, these are adjunct treatments and not replacements for an oncologist.

Recent studies continue to show increasing evidence that nondrug and nonsurgical therapies can be helpful when used along with conventional cancer treatments. Some of the complementary practices that have been scientifically proven to work are covered by insurance, so check with your provider.

In one study, acupuncture was tested in a group of breast cancer patients who were treated with chemotherapy that caused nausea. Those who were given five days of acupuncture, which is the stimulation of specific points along the body using thin needles or the application of heat pressure or laser light, had one-third fewer episodes of nausea than those who were treated only with antinausea medications such as lorazepam and diphenhydramine. Self-administered acupressure, where patients press on certain points, such as the PC6 on the wrist (without the use of needles), has also proved helpful in some cases.

Acupuncture works by correcting imbalances in the body's natural flow of energy through channels known as meridians; it does not always involve being stuck like a porcupine with numerous needles. Practitioners say there are more than 400 acupuncture points all over the body, so stimulating points along these channels helps balance or correct any deficiencies or blockages.

Research using MRIs has shown that when you place a needle at certain acupuncture points, areas of the brain light up. The stimulated areas that are associated with our emotions release a flood of endorphins and dopamine that act as painkillers and mood enhancers.

Finding the PC6 Point

The "PC6 point" is said to relieve nausea, upset stomach, motion sickness, carpal tunnel, and headaches. If you are experiencing any of these symptoms, try this DIY acupressure. Turn your hand so your palm is facing up and find the area between the tendons three finger widths from the base of the wrist. Massage the area for four to five seconds or longer as needed.

Get the Massage

A study with approximately 1,300 cancer patients found that massage improved their pain scores by 40 percent and that improvements lasted for hours and sometimes days afterward. Like acupuncture and acupressure, gentle massage can help relieve pain caused by chemotherapy and radiation treatments. It often allows patients to take lower doses of medication, which can reduce the drug's side effects.

DIY Massage

Professional massages can be costly, especially if you live in a big city, so if you can't afford the full spa-treatment Monty, I recommend a 10-minute chair massage (done fully clothed and available at many nail salons for around $10 plus tip). Many cancer hospitals offer complementary medical treatments for patients, including massage, acupuncture, as well as yoga/meditation classes.

If you want a do-it-yourself massage, you can buy aromatic massage oils online (try mountainroseherbs.com) or at your local health food store. These special oils have therapeutic botanical properties and can be warmed up to enhance the massage experience. Test by putting a drop on your wrist before applying. Start with the crown of your head and work slowly out from there in circular strokes. Spend a couple of minutes massaging your entire scalp (home to many vital energy points). Don't forget your feet, which are filled with nerve endings that reflexologists (foot acupressurists) say are connected to essential organs.

6
DEM BONES: ORTHOPEDICS

· ·

Vicki Harrison suffered a crush injury from a 90-pound metal scaffolding bar that fell 10 feet onto her flip-flop-clad foot. After the accident, she developed a painful condition called reflex sympathetic dystrophy (RSD). This is her story.

Vicki Harrison's Story: RSD

"My journey with RSD began after my foot injury, causing symptoms that included extreme burning pain, swelling, and discoloration. The pain was so intense that I couldn't touch anything with my foot, including a blanket, bed sheet, or socks. This made it difficult for me to sleep at night or wear shoes. I'd have to shower on a stool with my foot underneath because water spray brought tears to my eyes! After the accident, all I could do was sit in my recliner and walk with crutches. I only went out in public when necessary for fear that someone or something might bump my foot.

My doctor gave me three sympathetic nerve block injections, which are a series of epidural steroid vaccinations done under anesthesia, to relieve my pain. There was little improvement. After the third nerve block injection, I was only able to lightly touch the foot in one area. I began searching the Internet for *any* other options for my RSD, which is where I learned about hyperbaric oxygen therapy. I found several HBOT facilities in my area, but none would even consider accepting me as a patient because HBOT was not an FDA-approved treatment for RSD.

My emotional roller coaster ride continued. I can't describe the frustration I felt at finding a possible solution only to be told I couldn't even try it! But I continued my search for someone, anyone, who would treat me. I became depressed at my doctor's recommendation that I take pain meds, creams, and nerve blocks to enable me to handle the pain. I was given little hope of full recovery. My long-term goal was getting my foot back to normal, as opposed to simply dealing with the pain. That's when I called Dr. Paul Harch's clinic in Louisiana.

Even though I live in Virginia my family strongly encouraged me to go. I was hesitant because of the cost, time away from home, and the uncertainty of results (Dr. Harch made it clear that there were no guarantees), but my husband insisted I give HBOT a try. At this point, I was frightened about the possibility of being in agony for the rest of my life. I spoke with the director at RSD Foundation, who suggested I try a new drug instead that was just being introduced onto the market, and he warned me about the expense and lack of positive results from HBOT. Despite this, my husband insisted that I try HBOT. It involved sacrifices from him and others in my family, including my sister, who took six weeks of leave from her job as a nurse to help me in New Orleans, and my brother-in-law, who drove us there from Virginia (a two-day drive). Because of the pain and swelling, flying was out of the question for me.

I have received a total of 32 HBOT treatments, the last one on October 30, 2014. No maintenance treatments have been necessary so far. After HBOT, I was able to walk, run (not fast or for long periods), dance, swim, camp, bike, canoe, garden, and cook—basically, anything I want to do. I can even fly again. I am currently working as a substitute school teacher. I have always lived an active lifestyle (I'm a retired dance instructor). I do have limited endurance, but whenever I begin to feel pain in my foot, I simply take a break and I'm ready to go soon after. I believe God chose to heal me through Dr. Harch and his staff, and thanks to HBOT, I now have my life back!"

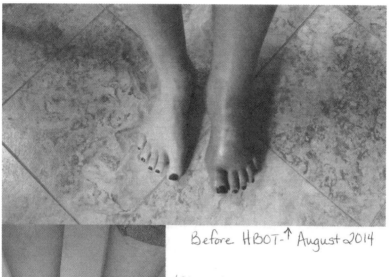

Before HBOT-↑ August 2014

After HBOT
January 2015 ←

Dr. Maxfield's Story: Joint Replacement

I can say from personal experience that hyperbaric oxygen therapy markedly improves healing after orthopedic surgery and gets patients back on their feet faster, whether it's an operation for the knee, hip, or back. I have had two hip replacements, and I was told by my surgeon that I could expect a six-week recovery. After getting HBOT before and after surgery, my recovery time was cut to only one week. HBOT is especially effective when treating orthopedic conditions because it stimulates the growth of new bone tissue that produces bone remodeling (the production of new cartilage), which speeds up the healing process.

Another Alternative to Back and Joint Surgery

Several years ago, my wife tripped over a poodle (yes, you read correctly), which brought on sciatica so severe that she needed crutches to get around. Her neurologist said that she would need six months of physical therapy and would probably have to undergo surgery.

That's when we learned about biomodulators, which provide electrical stimulation to the affected region, much like an updated version of acupuncture. It is extremely effective in treating back problems and injured joints. After just two biomdulator treatments, my wife was off her crutches. After six treatments, her sciatica was gone. The moral of this story: explore the alternatives before you get back surgery.

Rheumatoid Arthritis

Arthritis afflicts many of us as we age. It is an inflammation of the joints and the tissue surrounding them. Osteoarthritis, sometimes called degenerative joint disease or "wear and tear" arthritis, is the most common chronic condition of the joints affecting baby boomers 65 and older. In some cases, treating osteoarthritis patients with slightly increased hyperbaric pressure has been shown to relieve achy, arthritic joints. There have been a number of Russian studies on the benefits of hyperbaric oxygen therapy for rheumatoid arthritis. Rheumatoid arthritis is a chronic inflammatory disorder that is typically located in the small joints of your hands and feet. Unlike the "wear and tear" damage, rheumatoid arthritis affects the lining of your joints, causing a painful swelling that can eventually result in bone erosion and joint deformity. Rheumatoid arthritis is one of many forms of the disease where the immune system can attack the joint tissue as if it were a foreign object like a transplanted organ. In this case, HBOT can inhibit the self-destructive actions of the immune system.

I've also had excellent success in treating herniated discs and hip replacements with HBOT. In addition to my own experience, one of my patients was able to return to work within one week rather than the projected six-week recovery time after having a second hip replacement (the cement used to hold his prosthesis together had started to unglue).

Fibromyalgia

Fibromyalgia is a chronic pain syndrome that can be accompanied by other physical and mental conditions, including fatigue, cognitive impairment, irritable bowel syndrome, and sleep disturbance. "More than 90 percent of those diagnosed with the syndrome are women," according to Eshel Ben-Jacob, who was senior investigator at the Center for Theoretical Biological Physics at Tel Aviv University, Israel.

"Women who suffer from fibromyalgia benefit from a treatment regimen in a hyperbaric oxygen chamber," concluded Ben-Jacob, lead author of a clinical trial for women diagnosed with fibromyalgia. The painful condition improved in every one of the 48 women who completed two months of hyperbaric oxygen therapy. Brain scans of the women were taken before and after treatment, proving the theory that abnormal conditions in pain-related areas of the brain may be responsible for the syndrome. "Symptoms in about

70 percent of the women who took part in the study have to do with the interpretation of pain in their brains," Ben-Jacob explained. "They're the ones who showed the most improvement with hyperbaric oxygen treatment."

Scientists are still unsure of the syndrome's cause, although another recent study identified a possible RNA-based biomarker for its diagnosis.[1] (RNA stands for ribonucleic acid, a nucleic acid present in all living cells.) A variety of treatments from drugs to lifestyle changes have been tried to relieve patients' suffering with limited success.

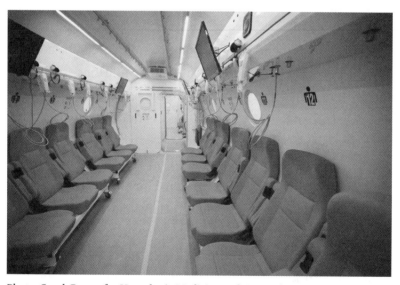

Photo: Sagol Center for Hyperbaric Medicine and Research.

Two 20-seat hyperbaric chambers at the Sagol Center for Hyperbaric Medicine and Research in Israel were used in a study to see if hyperbaric oxygen could help patients with fibromyalgia. Researchers at the Sagol Center and those at Tel Aviv University were studying posttraumatic brain injuries when they discovered that hyperbaric oxygen treatment could also help patients with fibromyalgia. "Patients who had fibromyalgia in addition to their concussion symptoms had complete resolution of the symptoms," said Dr. Shai Efrati, lead author of the study. One subject, an Oxford graduate student, developed fibromyalgia after suffering a traumatic brain injury in a train crash.

"The abnormalities in brain regions responsible for the chronic pain sensation in fibromyalgia patients can be triggered by different events," Dr. Efrati explained. "We have learned, for example, that when fibromyalgia is triggered by traumatic brain injury, we can expect complete resolution without any need for further treatment. However, when the trigger is attributed to other causes, such as fever-related diseases, patients will probably need periodic maintenance therapy."

The scientists noted the successful hyperbaric oxygen therapy enabled patients to drastically reduce or even eliminate their use of pain medications. "The intake of the drugs eased the pain but did not reverse the condition, while HBOT did reverse the condition," Dr. Efrati said of the findings, adding that they warrant further study. "The results are significant because, unlike current treatments offered for fibromyalgia patients, HBOT is not aiming for just symptomatic improvement but for the actual cause—the brain pathology responsible for the syndrome. It means brain repair, including neuronal regeneration, is possible even for chronic, long-lasting pain syndromes."[2]

HBOT and Sports

Both professional and amateur athletes alike have discovered the benefits of HBOT when it comes to recovering from sports injuries. The Canadian Canucks, for example, introduced HBOT for their injured hockey players, cutting the time players spent on the bench by half.

Those of us in the field have seen (and experienced firsthand) how HBOT can help speed up the healing process after sports surgeries. Dr. Harch, who tore a calf muscle several years ago before going on a ski trip, went immediately to his HBOT clinic after being injured. Within 48 hours, he was walking on his bad leg, and in five weeks, he was well enough to hit the slopes. He used HBOT yet again to repair his anterior cruciate ligament (ACL), another injury common to athletes. Dr. Harch had hyperbaric treatments before and after the ACL reconstruction surgery and, as a result, suffered no postop swelling and immediately regained 90 degrees of movement in his knee. "My surgeon was so amazed he just said, 'Keep doing whatever you're doing,'" Dr. Harch recalls.

Oxygen as Performer Enhancer

Three of the top United States cyclists in the 2006 Tour de France were reported to have used a special (and legal) method to boost their performance, according to an article published that year in the *New York Times*. They slept in altitude tents or altitude rooms that simulate the low-oxygen conditions of high altitude.

Cyclists Dave Zabriskie, George Hincapie, and Levi Lei-pheimer were among the athletes featured on the Colorado Altitude Training website, a company that makes tents known as hypoxic devices. "Runners, triathletes, skiers, rowers and the Philadelphia Flyers are among the elite athletes who es-pouse the virtues of the company's altitude simulation prod-ucts on the site," the article reports. "Some would like to ban the altitude tents and rooms as an unfair advantage be-cause the agency deemed the oxygen tents and rooms vio-lated the 'spirit of the sport.'"

The ramifications of banning these hypoxic devices, athletes and trainers told the *New York Times*, would be far-reaching, and many are upset that anyone would even consider putting the kibosh on this "natural" performance-enhancing technique. It would mean that the question of a performance booster moves from the use of drugs, like an-abolic steroids and human growth hormone, to something much more nebulous, such as oxygen.

Athletes who can afford it, and those whose schedules permit, often sleep in the mountains and travel to lower alti-tudes during the day to train. Others use the modern method: sleeping in altitude tents, which start at about $5,000 from Colorado Altitude Training. Some, like former NFL quarter-back Tim Tebow, use an oxygen chamber, while others con-vert a bedroom or building into livable oxygen chambers, spending anywhere from $25,000 to $1 million or more to convert an entire building.

Why do athletes use oxygen to improve their perfor-mance? As you now know, when the blood is full of oxygen, we consider this a 100 percent blood oxygen level. Most healthy athletes are probably around 95 or 97 percent blood oxygen level. As we expend energy, this level declines as the oxygen is consumed by our activity. When athletes train or compete, they must stop and catch their breath and reoxygenate their blood.

This is why some athletes want to increase their blood oxygen level *before* they compete. If they bring their oxygen level up to 99 or 100 percent, they will have more time before they need to stop and rest. When using HBOT prior to an event, athletes will notice a difference in how much energy they have before fatigue sets in. Getting an ample supply of oxygen will also flush out the lactic acid from the muscles, enabling athletes to function better.

Keep in mind that every athlete has a different body composition. One athlete may have a slightly higher blood oxygen level, for example, because he or she either is not exposed to secondhand smoke or lives and trains in a smog-free area. An athlete can also achieve a high blood oxygen level by training in high-altitude mountainous regions. Raising one's blood oxygen level from 97 percent to 99 percent can help shave off a second or two when biking, running, skiing, and myriad other sports.

If you are not fatigued or in need of oxygen, you may not notice an immediate benefit. Because every sport is unique, athletes need to develop a way to test their performance with and without oxygen. One way of measuring the benefits of HBOT when working out is to calculate your performance before and after hyperbaric oxygen. If you are a weightlifter, for example, count how many reps you can do lifting a dumbbell without oxygen. Then count the number of reps you can do after HBOT. You might notice an increase without feeling any effects on your body unless it is in need of oxygen.

A marathon runner can measure the time it takes before running out of gas and compare it to experiences with and without hyperbaric oxygen. A bike rider can calculate the speed and time difference while climbing a training hill. An athlete can also benefit from the increase in cognitive reasoning power. Typically an oxygenated athlete will be able to make faster and more accurate decisions while competing. A running back or quarterback carrying a football has to make quick decisions about where to zig and zag and when to throw the ball to avoid being tackled. The brain boost they get from HBOT can help them make these snap decisions.

Tennis Star Djokovic Sings HBOT's Praises

According to a 2016 article in the *Wall Street Journal*, some tennis players are using HBOT to get an advantage over their opponents. After winning a four-and-a-half-hour match at the Australian Open, tennis phenom Novak Djokovic beelined to an HBOT clinic called HyperMed located a few miles away from the stadium. The clinic has four "pods" where players get their postgame fix of 100 percent oxygen. At HyperMed, *WSJ* reporter Tom Perrotta says, Djokovic spent an hour in the pod after his five-setter against Gilles Simon. He also uses HBOT before matches, as he did for an hour prior to competing with Kei Nishikori.

Djokovic, known for his agile moves on the court, has used the pods for several years with the hope of aiding recovery and preventing injury, the article reports. Doubles star Mike Bryan also became a pod regular. His twin brother, Bob, tried it too, but just once. "It's great," Djokovic said. "It should get out there more, not just for athletes." Bryan added, "It just helps recovery. I felt a little better doing it."

Djokovic conceded that there is still a stigma about oxygen therapy, especially in Europe, where people believe that it gives athletes who use it a competitive edge. "It's very sensitive, especially in the European part of the world," he said. "I wish I can have this all over the place."

7

HEAD CASES: TRAUMATIC BRAIN INJURIES

. . . .

Dr. Steven Skaggs, a chiropractor based Joplin, Missouri, also operates an HBOT clinic for such conditions as multiple sclerosis, traumatic brain injury (TBI), diabetes, posttraumatic stress disorder, and Parkinson's disease. Below he recounts how his dying son taught him about the healing properties of HBOT.

Kayle's Story: TBI

"About four and a half years ago, I was piddling in the garage when my wife let out a blood-curdling scream. I ran upstairs where our 24-year-old son, Kayle, had died in his bedroom. His heart had stopped and he had no pulse. She immediately called 9-1-1 while I tried to get an airway clear for 13 minutes before EMS got there. I performed CPR and was able to get his heart rate back. Kayle, who had suffered from migraines that lasted for days, had been given a prescription medication that he had been using for a while to help with the headaches. The doctors said he had a sudden reaction to the drug that caused him to vomit and, because he was sleeping on his back, made him choke. He spent 11 days in a coma at the local intensive care unit in Joplin and then another 20 days in an ICU that specializes in traumatic brain injuries. After 31 days, where we never left his side, Kayle came out of his coma. We were ecstatic, but we knew if he woke up that he would have some brain damage or be in a vegetative state. The CAT scan that was done his first day demonstrated a 25 percent loss of the white matter inside his brain. His brain had shut down.

I spoke to my sister, who is a clinical psychologist, and she suggested hyperbaric oxygen treatment. I was unfamiliar with it, so I stayed up until 2 a.m. researching HBOT. Convinced that it would help Kayle, I begged our insurance company to pay for his hyperbaric treatments and sent studies proving that it works. They denied the request. I continued to stay up nights reading everything I could get my hands on about HBOT and faxed the information to the appeals committee. After eight months, the insurance company denied my appeal. That's when I got pissed off and purchased a hyperbaric chamber for my son. When Kayle first started HBOT, he couldn't tell you what a dime was or what he had for breakfast. He had hand tremors ever since the accident. After his first HBOT treatment, he came out and said, 'I'm hungry.' We all went out to eat and watched him feed himself. His tremor was gone and he could talk. I have had the privilege to watch this young man learn how to walk and talk again, and we have seen improvements ever since. Now we have two chambers in my office.

We had Kayle in the low-pressure chamber every day for an average of an hour and 10 minutes. He's had over 400 dives, and he still continues to improve and have maintenance treatments. Kayle is now 28 and a certified hyperbaric tech and safety director. He maintains my chambers and he's now looking for a job in other facilities. This experience has changed my entire view on the healing process. There are days we just break down and cry, but they are tears of joy."

Traumatic Brain Injuries

Traumatic brain injuries account for the majority of patients who seek HBOT treatments, and as you will read in this chapter, they have a wide range of causes, including accidents, weapon blasts, strokes, seizures, and concussions. In 1993, a patient suffering from a brain injury came to see me after a car accident that left him bedridden, incommunicative, and in need of 24-hour nursing care. Other doctors he had consulted told him he would never be able to leave his bed. His case was so severe that it required more than 300 hyperbaric treatments. By the end of his treatments in 2008, the man was walking with a cane, talking, and traveling with assistance. I'm pleased to report that he continues to improve each day.

Another patient I worked with was a child who also sustained a TBI after an auto accident. When I first saw her, she had a fractured leg and was unable to speak. Despite being admitted to a hospital equipped with a hyperbaric oxygen chamber, the doctors refused to give her HBOT treatments. When she was discharged, her parents took her to Dr. Richard Neubauer's clinic in Fort Lauderdale, Florida, where she was given 49 hyperbaric oxygen treatments. The HBOT allowed the girl to both walk and talk again. Ten years later, she is an honor student in high school.

Lori's Story: TBI

"I'm a single mom of two girls. My eldest daughter, Stephanie, graduated high school in 1999. A month later, Stephanie went on a horseback riding trip with some friends. We were living in Idaho at the time. Her foot got caught in the stirrup while she was dismounting so she could to pick wildflowers, and the horse took off into a full gallop, dragging her behind with her head hitting the ground. A helicopter had to transport Stephanie to the hospital because she was so far up in the mountains. By the time she got to the emergency room, she was in desperate need of surgery. She was just 18 at the time, and she had been planning to go to Europe. Needless to say, everything changed after that day.

She was unconscious and had surgery because both sides of her brain were filled with blood. The doctor was amazed that she was alive. She was in a coma for two and half months. When she finally opened her eyes, she didn't recognize us. There were so many people who came to visit that the hospital staff had to ask them to leave. Everyone was praying for her.

One of the male nurses in the ICU told me privately that he knew about an alternative treatment but he wasn't allowed to talk about it there, so he gave me a phone number for his wife. When I called, she told me about hyperbaric oxygen therapy. The other doctors and nurses told me I was wasting my money because we didn't know if HBOT would work, but I said, 'You're giving me no hope and now I have some hope.'

Stephanie was transferred from the hospital to a nursing home, where she was given no care at all. My family and friends took turns staying with her. We didn't want to leave her side. I had been working in the local school district, but I had to quit my job to become a full-time caregiver. Even the physical therapist at the nursing home said it was not the right place for her, so we took her to the brain injury unit in Spokane, Washington. The doctors there refused to give her HBOT even though they had the oxygen chambers because they said there wasn't enough information about it. That's when I decided to take her home.

She was in a wheelchair, and she couldn't hold her head up. Her eyes were open, but she wasn't reactive. The doctor said she wouldn't remember us if she woke up and that she would be a vegetable, which were the saddest words I had ever heard. The next part was a godsend. I was told the local newspaper wanted to interview me and that I should bring a picture of Steph. Two days later, I opened the paper and Stephanie was on the front page with our story inside. The reporter appealed to readers to donate money so we could get her to Canada for hyperbaric oxygen therapy, which was $150 a dive back then. A man gave us a van and carpenters installed a bed in it so she could lie down. My dad and I drove to Canada and rented out a basement suite.

She was semicomatose until February of 2000, when we finally took her to the hyperbaric oxygen clinic in Canada. She did 40 dives the first trip, and after a week, she waved at my father, who was watching her from outside the chamber. That day we had a party. From then on, she gradually became more alert. We would go for a month at a time for HBOT, come home for a few months, and return. She just continued to progress. Dr. Maxfield has been the consultant for her treatment. She literally had to relearn how to do everything. We would have a party each time she had a breakthrough, like tying her shoes or turning the pages of a book. It was like starting all over. She was in a wheelchair for about a year and then she started using a walker, then she walked by herself.

Stephanie is now 35 and we have since moved to North Dakota. I'd say she's had about 700 dives so far. We bought our own hyperbaric chamber so we can treat her at home at 1.5 levels. The last few times, she was able to get in and out of the chamber by herself. She was never able to do this before. I was amazed! But she's had a few setbacks. She was walking one day and just fell off the curb. We were told to cut back on the HBOT to see if she gets better and she did. But a week after that, she started falling again, so I talked to Dr. Maxfield to see if we should cut back on the oxygen treatments. Her progress is exciting, but we don't want to overdo it. Now she's become more stable again and we are beginning to see cognitive improvement such as word recognition.

Stephanie still lives with me, and she has a job at our church doing things around the office like shredding, vacuuming, and sending out bulletins. She recognizes all of us, and she has friends who she goes to the movies with. My advice to anyone going through a similar situation is to get to a hyperbaric chamber as soon as possible. It was six months before we got HBOT. Had we gotten her treatment sooner, she would have been that much better. I didn't know at the time. I fully believe that someday she will be healed. People say I'm crazy, but I'm a mom and I have to believe!"

Thousands Wrongly Placed in Nursing Homes

According to a 2016 article published in the *New York Times*, when patients in South Dakota seek help for serious yet manageable disabilities such as diabetes, blindness, or mental illness, they are funneled into nursing homes or long-term care facilities, much like the one where Stephanie was placed.

The Justice Department reported that thousands of patients were being held unnecessarily "in sterile, highly restrictive group homes." It deemed this practice a form of discrimination, making South Dakota the target of a federal effort to protect the civil rights of people with disabilities and mental illnesses. South Dakota is just one of many states that are under investigation for this kind of health care abuse, the article reports, with an estimated 250,000 working-age people who are needlessly living in nursing homes. With help, the Justice Department said, "Such people could live at home, hold hobs and lead productive lives. Instead they are confined and segregated from society." With wider acceptance of HBOT, this

will certainly lower the number of people unnecessarily placed in nursing homes and critical care facilitates.

Dan Greathouse's Story: Decompression Sickness

In 1991, Dan, a bright, dedicated 34-year-old junior
high school teacher from New Mexico, decided try
scuba diving. For someone who lives in a dry region,
this is an unusual form of recreation, but he went to
San Carlos, Mexico, to get properly trained and certified to be a diver. What happened after seems more
like fiction but is sadly all true. Due to a malfunction
in the "free flow regulator" attached to his oxygen
tank, coupled with having no diving buddy to assist
as he struggled to breathe, Dan ascended too quickly
from the dive, causing an air embolism to enter his
bloodstream. He didn't know it at the time, but Dan
would suffer from a severe case of decompression
sickness that wreaked havoc in his brain and his
life.

I spoke to Dan about his ordeal, which he chroni-
cles in his book, *Doc, I Want My Brain Back*. In our con-
versation, as in his book, Dan makes a compelling case
for the use of HBOT treatments for TBIs. Although
HBOT is universally accepted as a treatment for the
bends, even Dan's fellow divers failed to recognize his

condition. "The diving team didn't understand the effects brought on by the regulator malfunction and the high altitude of New Mexico," Dan explained. "Had I come up unconscious or with cramps in my arms and legs, they probably would have gotten me the proper treatment."

But instead of getting immediate hyperbaric therapy, his brain injury gradually robbed him of his memory, balance, and ability to think, walk, or play music. He was misdiagnosed by more than 30 medical professionals before receiving HBOT treatments that finally cured him, but his journey to recovery was a long, tortuous, and often painful one that nearly caused him to take his own life. Prior to his recovery, Dan committed himself to a mental hospital after planning suicide.

"After a few weeks in that hospital, I was handcuffed and taken to the San Juan detention center for a week," Dan recalls. "They wanted to have me evaluated for the state institution and, coincidentally, a woman from my neighborhood who was out race walking was brutally murdered and the police were convinced that I had done it. I looked similar to the picture of the suspect. Not one of my next of kin was notified that I was taken from the mental facility to jail. All I could do in my cell was shuffle back and forth and mutter 'God help me!'"

But Dan's parents eventually intervened and made provisions for him to be transferred to another mental hospital, where he was improperly drugged with psychotropic medications, an unwise course for some-one who was also a recovering alcoholic and had been three years sober. At the time, he said, many of his friends and family "wrote him off as a mental case." His parents and brother, however, continued taking him to see doctors in the hope of treating his decompression sickness. Time and again, he was told that HBOT was either quackery or too risky.

But Dan did get several HBOT sessions in New Mexico, which, sadly, did nothing because the doctors there were unfamiliar with the dosage and number of treatments necessary to treat his brain injury. "They were toying around with the pressure and the time, trying to squeeze the bubbles out of my brain. But by that time I had brain damage. They even spoke to Dr. Paul Harch on the phone, who explained to them that he had worked with divers who had delayed treatment and he even gave them the correct protocol. They just laughed him off. They thought more than three oxygen treatments was dangerous. Had they followed Dr. Harch's suggestions, I would have gotten better."

Dan finally decided to go to Dr. Harch's clinic in Louisiana.

"I was given brain scans that proved I had gotten decompression sickness, just as I had suspected, and that I wasn't crazy after all! As a recovering alcoholic, I had to get off the medication I was on at the mental hospital, so I was in detox until my body was clean.

I started with two HBOT treatments a day. I probably had a total of 100 treatments in all. In addition to the HBOT, I had physical therapy, meetings with social workers, and neuropsychological testing.

After a week or two of treatments, I got up one night to use the bathroom and I didn't have to hold onto anything for balance. I couldn't sleep the rest of the night because I was so excited. I started writing in my notebooks, which I couldn't do before without struggling! It was like turning on a light switch. I finally got my old life and brain back!

I am now fully recovered and in my fifth year as president of the Texas Educational Diagnostic Association, where I treat children with learning and intellectual disabilities. I've found my true calling as a result of my horrible experience. I play music again and I'm in a local band. I went back to the clinic around Christmas to get booster treatments for about a week, but I haven't had any HBOT since. My message to people who are told that there is nothing that can be done for their TBI is to find a reputable, experienced doctor who does hyperbaric oxygen therapy. Above all, never give up!"

Curt Allen Jr.'s Story: TBI

Another remarkable case involved a young man named Curt Allen Jr., a 17-year-old who got into a high-speed car accident in 2004, where he sustained severe traumatic brain injury. Curt, who was in a coma at the scene of the accident, underwent brain surgery to relieve pressure and, later, was placed in the ICU in critical condition. After one month, he was transferred to a brain injury rehabilitation center in Southeast Louisiana where he remained for three months.

During these three months, he made such minimal progress that he was discharged. The day before he left this center, his mother attended a local church where she asked the priest to request that the congregation pray for her son's recovery. After the priest fulfilled this request during mass, Mrs. Allen was approached by a physician, a patient of Dr. Harch's, who had received low-pressure HBOT years earlier for a stroke and subsequent traumatic brain injury.

So Curt's mom brought him to see Dr. Harch, who first evaluated him in October 2004 at his clinic. At the time, Curt was so badly brain damaged he couldn't lift his head, talk, or eat on his own. He was confined to a wheelchair. But after three months of HBOT treatments, Curt could lift his head and smile, By April 2005, he was using a walker, talking, and eating without a feeding tube. Two months later, after his 90th HBOT, he is walking unaided, talking, and eating normally. You can see a video of Curt's astounding recovery after four months of HBOT treatments on www.HBOT.com.

Jody James's Story: Epilepsy and TBI

"Our son, Joshua, had his first epileptic seizure when he was seven years old. He would have about two or three seizures a month. He was never incapacitated by the seizures, so he went to mainstream schools. He was even considered to be a gifted student in the fifth grade. We managed to have a relatively normal life with the antiseizure medication. Everything was fine until September 2014, when he went out to dinner with some friends. That night he had a seizure that caused him to fall down and hit his head. His friends called us to let us know they had taken him to the local emergency room.

The doctors did a CT scan and saw some internal bleeding, so he was transferred to another hospital. He was asked the mental competency questions—day, year, president's name, and so on—and he was able to answer all the questions, but 15 minutes later he couldn't. He squeezed my hand as if to say, 'What's happening to me, Mom?' I could see the fear in his eyes.

When Josh was 25, he had several surgeries, including one where 120 electrodes were attached to his brain to find the source of the seizures so doctors could remove the portion of his brain that was causing them. After that, he was seizure-free for nearly 10 years! He was able to live a completely normal life—walking, talking, and doing everything but driving. Then, in

2013, he started to have a seizure every two to three months, despite being able to live a normal life.

Back he went to the hospital, where he had six more operations over the course of 52 days, including one where surgeons removed a piece of his skull and put in shunts (used for water on the brain) and tubes. At that point, we were worried that Josh would be a vegetable. I happened to have a friend who worked as a nurse in that hospital. She confessed to me later that the team never thought Josh would survive. We were in denial. In addition to dealing with all these surgeries and treatments, we had to negotiate with the insurance companies to find out what was covered and what wasn't.

At that point, our lives consisted of mostly shuttling him back and forth from the hospital to a rehab facility due to various complications. He was bedridden and on a feeding tube. We had home health benefits, so we had a nurse and three therapists coming in a few days a week.

Dr. Skaggs, who lives in our town of Joplin, Missouri, called to talk to me about HBOT treatments for Josh. I told him I'd do some research on it, and we also asked our neurologist about HBOT. He said, 'There have been some good results, but it's not part of our protocol.' All the doctors we spoke to about it said the same thing. I finally called Dr. Skaggs's back to say I wanted to try it. He said, 'I was wondering when you were going to call me.'

Dr. Skaggs came to our house to talk to us because it was difficult for us to leave our bedridden son. At the time, my husband, who runs his own mechanics shop, and I hadn't been out to dinner for a year. Dr. Skaggs and his son, Kayle, came over and talked to us about a plan for Josh.

We started the HBOT treatments in April 2015. Josh needed to be lifted into the chamber. He was in a wheelchair, and he could barely talk. Now we do 10 days on and 10 days off for a little over an hour. After about 40 treatments, Josh did a swallow test with table food, and he passed with flying colors! There was a speech therapist and five other health care professionals at the rehab center watching Joshua swallow, and they attributed his success to HBOT.

We've removed his feeding tube, and he's talking a little, saying, 'Hi Mom,' 'Hi Dad,' 'Thanks,' 'Yes,' and 'No.' I told the speech therapist that my goal is to be able ask him if he is cold or hungry. All of his therapists are convinced that he understands everything. He has now had over 100 HBOT treatments, and he is making phenomenal progress. So far, we have achieved another goal, which is getting him out of his wheelchair. In April 2016, he walked for the first time with the help of parallel bars!"

Carol Lewin's Story: Epilepsy and Ataxia Telangiectasia

"Jimmy had his first epileptic seizure when he was about six months old. They were mild, persistent seizures of unknown origin. We tried one or two medicines that made him lethargic. My husband, who happened to work in DC in the same field as one of Dr. Maxfield's daughters, was introduced to HBOT through her. She said, 'You've got to take your son to see my father.' The more we learned about oxygen hyperbaric therapy, the more it made sense to us.

So we took him down to Florida for HBOT when he was just over two years old. I sat with him in a monoplace chamber, which was actually kind of a relaxing, and Jimmy had no problem with it at all. (My skin benefited greatly from being in the chamber as well!) We had about 40 one-hour treatments each day for a month. After a few weeks, Jimmy was more alert and we saw some marked improvements, including fewer seizures, although he was still developmentally delayed.

He had a good long-term period for years afterward, and we continued to go for maintenance treatments once a week at a clinic closer to our home in Virginia. He went to public school, and he could do most normal childhood activities, although he was wobbly. He later went to a special needs school in high school, which worked well for him.

Unfortunately, he has since been given another diagnosis of ataxia telangiectasia (AT), which is neurological degenerative disease similar to muscular dystrophy. AT affects his short-term memory and muscle control by causing brain cells to die out.

Our thinking was that if we give him HBOT, his brain cells would become saturated with oxygen, which would have a positive result for both of his conditions.

We talked to him about going back into the chamber after his AT diagnosis but stopped doing HBOT when Jimmy got older and decided he didn't want to do it anymore. We have to respect his wishes because he is a young adult now, even though we know the HBOT would help him. But his baseline treatment allowed us to take him off of most his medications except for a mild dose of one old drug.

If we hadn't had someone like Dr. Maxfield give us such good treatments at an early age, I don't know if Jimmy would have had such good results. As far as his AT is concerned, he is ahead of what is expected for someone with this disease. The prognosis is that AT patients don't live past age 20, and he's now 23, so that's a blessing. In the past four months, he's gotten another troubling diagnosis of esophageal cancer. I'm exploring getting him back on HBOT for his surgery to remove the tumor because I know that it helps in wound healing. A nurse gave me some good advice about looking into a multichamber where I can go in with him. I think he would be emotionally calmer if I was there with him.

In a day and age when so many medications are available, many of which have some negative side effects, hyperbaric oxygen is a safe, noninvasive alternative for so many people. It worked for my son, and I believe it can help others as well."

Understanding Epilepsy

Epilepsy, also known as seizure disorder, is a neurological condition caused by recurring disruptions of electrical communication in the brain. These disruptions are called seizures. Not everyone who has a seizure has epilepsy, but according to the Epilepsy Foundation, one in 26 people in the United States will develop epilepsy at some time in their life. A diagnosis of epilepsy will result after two or more unprovoked seizures have occurred more than 24 hours apart. A seizure is considered unprovoked if there is no underlying condition or trigger that may have caused it, such as a stroke, infection, or head injury.

Symptoms of Epilepsy

Seizures cause a variety of symptoms ranging from a blank stare to sudden uncontrollable movements that are often accompanied by a loss of or altered state of consciousness. Most seizures last for just two minutes or less. Some seizures will cause a person to suddenly collapse or fall to the ground. Generalized seizures affect the whole brain and are most commonly associated with convulsions or jerking and stiffening of muscles in the head, back, arms, or legs. Other symptoms include loss of consciousness, rhythmic jerking, or falling. With some types, loss of bladder control and tongue biting are also possible symptoms.[1]

Valerie Greene's Story: Stroke

Valerie Greene became an advocate of hyperbaric oxygen therapy after suffering a massive stroke at the age of 31. She lost most of her hearing, and doctors told her she might never walk or talk again. Today there is practically nothing she *can't* do. Valerie has inspired thousands of survivors around the world by telling her story and offering a go-to resource of information on HBOT and other treatments on her website, www.bcenter.com. This is her story.

"After my stroke, I couldn't talk and I was paralyzed from the neck down. All I could do was scream. I learned how to say one word, which was 'help!' I learned about HBOT from my high school boyfriend who came to visit me at the hospital. He said, 'I'm going to take you to a doctor who can help you.'

I didn't think much about it at the time, but, sure enough, the day I was released he came with his pickup truck to take me in my wheelchair to an HBOT clinic here in Orlando. I remember the doctor so well with his cowboy boots and beer belly. He said, 'I can help you, but you have to go out of the United States because we're not allowed to practice this therapy for what you have.'

I told him I didn't care if I had to eat bananas upside down, just help get me out of this wheelchair. It was expensive, and I wasn't making as much money back then, but I bought my plane ticket and went. I don't want to say where because I'm not sure who's operating the clinic now. The oxygen tank was really rudimentary compared to what we have now. It was homemade, and it had a tiny window where I could look out. They slid me in and riveted the sides shut. Despite this crazy-looking machine, I felt really relaxed.

I had two oxygen treatments daily for 40 days—once in the morning and once in the evening. There was a TV monitor on the outside and only one video, *The Terminator*, in Spanish, which I watched over and over again! The first thing I said after coming out of the chamber was '*Hasta la vista*, baby,' but I was able to talk! I could also wiggle my toes and my left foot, which had been paralyzed. When I got back home to Florida, Dr. Maxfield and Dr. Neubauer took over my treatment, and they were instrumental in my recovery. I went from the wheelchair, to a walker, to a three-pronged cane, to a single cane, to walking alone. That took about two years.

Having a stroke has changed me forever. Now I see it as a gift because I have been called as a messenger to help other survivors. I said a prayer when I was in the hospital, 'God, if you just give me my voice back, I promise I will never stop telling my story.' When I got my voice back, I fulfilled my promise. Now I hear about people's experiences with HBOT from all over the world. When people ask me about the one thing that helped me most, I'd have to put HBOT at the top of my list. I always give credit first and foremost to God, of course.

I'm 52 now, and if you look at me, you'd never know I had a stroke. My recovery was a remarkable one, but it takes time. Don't expect to immediately get up and walk. You have to be patient. Don't push it. You need to shower your body with love, comfort, and rest. I used to tell my left side to comfort the right side by saying, 'You're doing great—you can do this!' Your body heals most when it's resting, and where better than in an oxygen tank? The oxygen will help your brain cells regenerate, and it laid the foundation for my recovery. It's like a fog has been lifted. I can think, remember, hear, see, and speak better. There are certain things I can't do like run, and I have a little weakness on my left side.

My goal, which I share with Dr. Maxfield, is to get HBOT where it should be in this country. I want to build a center in Orlando where stroke survivors can receive all their treatments in one place. It would be called the Bcenter (Be Well at the Bcenter). There will be a program where people are taught how to recover. It can be a lifelong process, but I am a beacon of hope. This too shall pass, if you let it!"

What Is a Stroke?

A stroke occurs when blood flow to part of the brain is interrupted, and the lack of oxygen and nutrients causes brain cells to die. There are various ways this can happen. Blocked arteries or blood clots are the most common cause of stroke, affecting 700,000 Americans annually. Blood clots arise from inflamed arterial plaques and from an unhealthy heart. When blood clots break off and travel in the bloodstream to the brain, they can become lodged in an artery. If this happens, the area of the brain supplied by that artery will die.

Another cause of stroke is a ruptured blood vessel in the brain. This can cause what's called a "cerebral hemorrhage," or bleeding within the brain. Uncontrolled hypertension is the most common cause of cerebral hemorrhage. Abnormalities in cerebral blood vessels, including aneurysms (an abnormal ballooning of the vessel wall) and arteriovenous malformations (an abnormal collection of blood vessels), can also cause bleeding in the brain.

Some warnings of a ruptured aneurysm include a severe headache that comes on suddenly and reaches its maximum intensity in just seconds. Stroke survivors often describe this abrupt onset headache as feeling as if they were hit on the head with a bat. The headache is sometimes accompanied by a stiff neck that comes from blood tracking around the brain and down the spinal cord. If you are experiencing the above symptoms, seek immediate medical attention.

The symptoms of stroke depend on what part of the brain is deprived of blood flow. If a motor pathway is affected, for example, the ability to move will be impaired. If language areas are deprived of blood flow, you might have trouble understanding what people are saying, appear confused, or have difficulty talking. In some cases, people might not even be aware that they are having a stroke because the part of the brain that perceives changes in the body is impaired.

Get Help F-A-S-T

An easy way to remember and respond to the warning signs for a stroke is to think FAST. The acronym stands for

Facial drooping
Arm weakness
Speech difficulty
Time to call 9-1-1

The American Academy of Neurology, the American College of Emergency Physicians, and the American Stroke Association say the following five symptoms might indicate that you or someone you know is having or has had a stroke:

1. **Walk.** Is your balance off? Are you dragging one leg? Are you veering to one side?
2. **Talk.** Is your speech slurred? Are you using the appropriate words? (Do your words make sense?) Does one side of your mouth droop down?
3. **Reach.** Is one side of your body weak or numb? Can you raise both your arms up together? Does one arm being to fall down? Can you squeeze your fingers with each hand? Is one hand weaker than another?
4. **See.** Is your vision all or partly lost? Do you see double?
5. **Feel.** Do you have a severe headache that peaked within seconds? If you normally have headaches, is this headache different from the others and feel like the worst headache you've ever had?

If you have these symptoms and think you are having a stroke, it is imperative to get to a hospital as soon as possible. Although the risk of stroke increases as we get older, it can occur at any age, even in children.

More Hope for Stroke Survivors

A new study released in April 2016, found that 91 percent of people given a stent retriever along with proper medication within two and a half hours of the stroke had little or no disability. After five and a half hours, 41 percent had similar results.

Healing Our Wounded Warriors

Hyperbaric oxygen alleviated PTSD symptoms secondary to a brain injury in 5 out of 5 peer-reviewed clinical trials.

—Xavier Figueroa, PhD, president, The Brain Health and Healing Foundation, Seattle, Washington

In my work at veterans hospitals, I've seen numerous soldiers who were told that their posttraumatic stress disorder (PTSD) symptoms were purely psychological—this is simply not the case. Desperate for some kind of medical treatment to relieve their depression and pain, we gave them brain scans that showed the precise areas where their brain

damage occurred. We also did extensive psychological testing and came to the same conclusion—PTSD is a physical
condition.

A 2006 article titled "Military TBI during the Iraq and Afghanistan Wars," by Dr. Deborah Warden (published in the
Journal of Head Trauma Rehabilitation), confirmed what many
of us in the field have known for years: TBI is the most common cause of brain injuries among soldiers, and it should be
treated along with PTSD.

One such veteran, a 40-year-old male with PTSD, complained of headaches, pain, dizziness, and depression. He
tried to commit suicide three times. He was unable to read,
so a psychologist had to read questions to him. Although he
lived in a small community, he had to use a GPS when driving
because he would forget where he was going. His first SPECT
scan showed severe damage in nearly all parts of his brain.
After 40 HBOT treatments, we scanned him again and the
new images found renewed activity in the brain. His psychological evaluation also revealed that his depression was lifting and his spirits were improving. Not only did his memory
get sharper after HBOT, but he was able to read again and
drive a car using his own navigational skills.

Another patient I worked with, who was 32, had both TBI
and PTSD. His symptoms included a loss of balance whenever he closed his eyes. He could not get up in the middle of
the night to use the bathroom without turning a light on. He
suffered from severe headaches, as well as tinnitus (a ringing or buzzing in the ears). Not surprisingly, a SPECT scan
revealed that he had extensive brain damage. After 40 HBOT

treatments, we did another scan and discovered an increase in normal brain activity. He no longer had dizzy spells, headaches, or ringing in the ears, and he is now living a happy, symptom-free life.

Battle-scarred soldiers like these often experience something similar to those who suffer from caisson disease, the decompression sickness that was described by Dan Greathouse. A study conducted in Budapest, Hungary, showed that people with caisson disease have an increased risk of suicide much like soldiers with TBI or PTSD.

Raymond Crallé, a respected physical therapist and HBOT clinician who operates the Oxygen Rescue Care Center of America in Del Ray, Florida, has been successfully treating veterans with PTSD and blast injuries. His HBOT treatments for vets are paid for by the Veterans Administration's Choice Program (see the Resources chapter). Crallé wrote the following about his work treating a marine with TBI, for whom I read SPECT scans, in a 2016 article published in the *New England Journal of Medicine*: "This case study documents what occurred to one veteran diagnosed with PTSD after multiple blast exposures; he had attempted suicide and was receiving treatment with psychotropic medications. After 40 hyperbaric oxygen therapy treatments (HBOT) and comprehensive physical therapy, the comparison of pre- and post-treatment neuropsychological tests, and SPECT brain scans documented significant improvement in cognitive function, motor skills, mental health state, and quality of life."

Another patient of Crallé's, Colonel Washington Sanchez Jr., is a Purple Heart Artillery Battalion Commander who served in Vietnam. He is currently undergoing HBOT and has had 20 dives as of this writing. I am interpreting the results of his SPECT scans as well. This is his story.

Colonel Washington Sanchez Jr.'s Story

"I am chairman of the Florida Veterans Foundation in Tallahassee, which funds HBOT treatments for veterans. This includes transportation and hotel costs for those coming from out of town. I served two tours in Vietnam. The first one was in 1965 when I was 22. I was a second lieutenant with an infantry company on a search-and-destroy mission. I lasted 90 days before we were ambushed. A number of soldiers were killed and wounded. I was one of the fortunate ones to survive with two bullets in my left leg. But I lay on the battlefield for quite a while before help came. Because I wasn't as bad off as some of the other soldiers, I was on a stretcher in a field hospital overnight before a doctor came to treat me. There just weren't enough beds. I was given morphine for the pain while I waited. Luckily the bullets didn't shatter any bones. I returned to Vietnam as a commander from 1968 to 1970.

It took about 50 years before I was able to talk about what happened there. At various times, I had flashbacks and nightmares and didn't know why. We didn't know about PTSD, or Agent Orange, or any of that stuff back then. I just ignored them and the VA did too because they didn't want us to submit for disability benefits. We had to prove that we suffered from PTSD, so I spoke to psychologists and got 30 percent coverage. It wasn't the money I wanted; I just wanted to get better. I worked myself ragged so I could avoid thinking about the war. I volunteered a lot and did some real estate work to keep myself busy. I tried to stay ahead of the PTSD.

Once I met Ray Crallé, my life changed. He told me that he could help my PTSD with HBOT. It turned out my headaches and PTSD was caused by the large artillery that we would fire all day long. The guns made so much noise that the bunkers I slept in would move from one side to the other. That's how much vibration was created by the blasts. I now know that these blasts were the cause of my TBI because experimental data has shown that machine and antitank fire creates air bubbles in the blood that damage the brain.

I read about oxygen hyperbaric therapy and decided I wanted to try it for myself before I recommended it to any other veterans. HBOT has done two things for me: my disposition has improved, and I'm not in pain anymore. I had 23 treatments last year. Before the HBOT, I had a SPECT scan taken, and lo and behold, it clearly showed that I had TBI. I'm now getting an additional 10 HBOTs. I had another SPECT scan after my treatments, and I can see the changes in my brain. The change has been phenomenal. I had knee pain that would cause me to scream whenever it touched against something. Now I don't have any pain in my knee or body. I've had to deal with this for more than 50 years, so you can imagine what it feels like not to be in pain! I couldn't garden or walk for long distances. Now I can walk five miles a day. I have more energy, and I no longer huff and puff.

It's amazing that I've survived the pain and TBI for so long. I'm 74 and I think about what my life would have been like had I done HBOT in my 20s! I've had suicidal thoughts in the past, but I never attempted anything. I was quick to anger with my first wife and at work, but I kept it under control. Now I can enjoy my relationships with my two wonderful kids and my second wife.

I'm now working with an Iraqi War veteran who is struggling with PTSD. He tried to kill himself by lying in the middle of the road. When he woke up, he saw his leg a hundred feet in front of him. The person who ran him over didn't stop, but when a lady stopped to help him, he asked her if she had a gun so he could shoot himself. He had migraines, anger problems, and drug and alcohol addiction. I'm hoping we can get him a few treatments starting tomorrow. He's trying to stay clean and sober. The foundation is paying for his treatment.

It's sad that the VA hospitals are refusing to pay for HBOT treatments for veterans with PTSD. We have hundreds of thousands of veterans who have been diagnosed with TBI and PTSD, and the only treatment they are approved for are pills. Some veteran once said the VA gives us a second chance to die. I knew a guy who was taking 18 pills a day. I told him once he gets a few HBOTs, he won't need any of those pills anymore."

Note: See www.floridaveteransfoundation.org for a video on the use of HBOT for TBI. Go to "What We Do" and click on "Hyperbaric Oxygen Therapy."

Save Our Soldiers

According to the US Department of Defense, more than 350,000 soldiers have been diagnosed with TBI between 2000 and 2015, many of them from blast exposures. The actual number might be higher due to the fact that many service men and women are reluctant to report or seek treatment for a condition that is not physically visible. This disturbing statistic is probably the reason 25 veterans commit suicide each day

Scientists suspect that explosive blasts affect the brain in the same way concussions and the bends do. These kinds of injuries can cause what's called chronic traumatic encephalopathy (CTE), a serious condition found in both soldiers and football plays that can lead to

irrational or violent behavior, depression, and
suicide. At the moment, CTE can only be diagnosed when an autopsy is performed.

Lieutenant Mike's Story: Migraines

"Ten days after Katrina, I came back from Baghdad.
That's when my migraines started. The migraines were
so painful that I was unable to work, and I was forced
to live off my military pension and social security,
which I took early. The migraines kept getting worse
and worse. I'd get a pounding headache from the top
of my head to the back of my eyeball in my skull up to
three times a week. It felt like the left side of my head
was being crushed by a vice. I'd wind up on the floor in
the fetal position.

I'm used to a lot of pain; I've broken ankles, and
I've been beat up pretty good a few times. That kind
of pain goes away. But the migraines feel like you're
being tortured. They'd last from 4 hours to 48 hours.
They would wake me up out of a dead sleep early in
the morning. I'm allergic to MSG, which also gives me
headaches, but nothing like the migraines.

I tried to get the Veterans Administration to give me
medication, but the first drug I was given was a generic
version of methadone. I remember lying on my back in
pain and taking the pills. My wife asked, 'Are you OK?'

I said, 'No, but I don't care.'

She looked up the name on the bottle and screamed. I am a recovering alcoholic, so the last thing I need are addictive drugs. We flushed the pills and that was that. They also tried giving me muscle relaxers and other pain medications, but none of them relieved the migraines. I finally got an appointment with a physician at the VA who wanted to give me Botox injections in my left temple. It relieves the symptoms for six to eight weeks, but the side effects can include muscle and face paralysis, stroke, or death. I said, 'I'll take the headaches, thank you.'

One of my soldiers suffered the same headaches and had PTSD and a lot of other issues. He was on about 10 different medications that the VA had given him. We didn't see him for six months. When he came back, he had lost weight, his demeanor was pleasant, and his headaches were gone. He told me he had been given hyperbaric oxygen treatments from the Wounded Warrior Project. He was off most of his medications, and he was able to work as a supervisor at a security company, coach Little League, and go back to school. His life had turned around completely.

I said, 'I want what you got.'

That's when I first saw Dr. Harch. I was evaluated for hours. My wife went with me because sometimes I couldn't get the words out of my mouth. My mental capacity was so diminished. I had been in three

near-fatal truck wrecks where my head hit the wind-
shield. At Fort Hood, I slipped and fell and I had to
crawl back to my room. I had multiple mild concussions within a year's time, two of them in one night. I
got SPECT scans taken, and you could see the difference in blood flow between the right and left sides of
my brain. My left side was shriveled up like a bunch
of dried grapes.

I would do whatever it took, including sell my
house, to get relief. I started the hyperbaric therapy a few days after Labor Day in 2014. At about the
13th treatment, I stopped getting migraines. It was
September 23, 2014. I wrote down the day so I'd
never forget it. As of today, it's been 1,001 days in a
row that I haven't felt that bone-crushing headache.
After the HBOT treatments, my scans showed that
my brain was normal again. I've never been a POW,
but I feel like I've been released from prison. My co-
ordination and memory also improved. My hand used
to quiver. I couldn't even walk a straight line. I used to
get a swelling in my right leg, and that went away
and hasn't returned. My energy level is up. After 40
treatments, I was done. I went back once again when
I broke my wrist, and I got five treatments before
and after my surgery and I barely have a scar. I still
count the days that I'm migraine-free. I like to say
that HBOT gives hope for the hopeless."

More Evidence of TBI in Veterans

A 2016 study by the Veterans Affairs Puget Sound Health Care System and UW Medicine at the University of Washington, Seattle, examined the effects of repeated explosions on veterans with mild traumatic brain injury.

The study found the more blasts one is exposed to, the more the brain is affected. Researchers tested 41 veterans with a history of mild TBI. They found the impacts were most noticeable in the lower regions of the cerebellum, the area of the brain that sits right at the base of the skull in the back of the head. The cerebellum coordinates movement, helps control mood and cognitive functions, and helps multitask. Veterans with mild TBI often report depression, irritability, impulsivity, and problems managing certain tasks.

American Association for Hyperbaric Awareness Meets with the Department of Defense

Thomas Fox, a certified HBOT clinician who lives and practices in Montreal, Canada, used to fly a medevac where he rescued soldiers in the battlefield, including Major Ben Richards, who was injured in an IED blast.

"After that incident, Major Richards had a steep decline in his IQ, which used to be 148," Fox says. "He was almost suicidal until he got HBOT." In 2004, Fox went to the White House as a member of the American Association for Hyperbaric Awareness task force to explain how hyperbaric oxygen treatment can and should be used to help our troops. In 2009, he briefed the Secretary of the Army about HBOT. Another member of the team was Brigadier General (R) Thomas P. Maney, who was in the Florida National Guard. He, too, had been injured by an IED, which resulted in a complete loss of memory. After hyperbaric treatments, he is now a sitting judge.

"We routinely go to DC to discuss this with the government," says Fox, "and we will continue to go until it recognizes HBOT's benefits for our wounded warriors and the VA covers the costs of treatments."

Military's Flawed Tests

First the good news: the US military has conducted tests on the value of HBOT for soldiers. Now the bad news: the tests are deeply flawed and the results are inaccurate. In contrast, a review of five large studies done on the use of hyperbaric oxygen in veterans suffering from TBI and PTSD by researchers Xavier Figueroa and James Wright of the Brain Health and Healing Foundation in Seattle, found symptoms from both conditions improved dramatically after HBOT. The results, which were published in a 2016 issue of *Neurology*, were a direct contradiction to the studies conducted by the Department of Defense, the VA, and the army.

"The military studies were poorly done because researchers used low-level oxygen concentrations that lessened the therapeutic effects," Figueroa said. "There was no one trained in HBOT conducting the studies," he continued. "It's like giving someone a single pill dose instead of three. There will be a difference in the effects based on the dosage. They were using inadequate oxygen dosing."

Another flaw was in the use of air under pressure, which the military researchers mistakenly called a placebo. The fact is air under pressure is not a placebo because there is a rise in oxygen levels in the blood when air pressure is increased. The results, therefore, did not show a significant difference between the placebo group versus the one receiving HBOT.

The failure to understand that air under pressure is not a placebo goes back many years to a Canadian study on treatment for cerebral palsy using HBOT, which produced the same results. Once again, my experience, and that of my colleagues in the field, is that HBOT is extremely effective in treating cerebral palsy.

The bottom line is that more studies need to be done by the military (and academic institutions) with the proper supervision of clinicians and doctors who are certified in hyperbaric medicine. For starters, SPECT brain scans can now be used to show the difference between traumatic brain injuries and PTSD. Patients with TBI or blast exposures will show areas of *decreased* localization on the SPECT brain scan, as opposed to those with pure PTSD, which will show some *increased* localization on the scan in certain areas of the brain. The ability to correctly interpret these scans is critical when deciding on treatment protocols for these two separate conditions. It is especially important for veterans who are repeatedly told by the VA that their symptoms are purely psychological.

Jennifer Crichton's Family Story: Concussions

"My family has experienced amazing healing miracles from HBOT, and we have met many others who have as well that I want to shout it from the mountain tops!

My two daughters and I had HBOT treatments starting in 2013. My oldest, Emily, then 22, was recommended to Dr. Harch by a nurse practitioner Emily was seeing for her 'developmental delays.' The nurse had a son with autism who spoke for the first time after having hyperbaric oxygen treatments. When we learned the HBOT clinic was outside of New Orleans, my husband and I were hesitant. We live in Maine and New Orleans is 1,800 miles away. But we decided to go with our hostile, challenging daughter nevertheless. When we saw Dr. Harch, he told me Emily's problems stemmed from her birth trauma. I had been in labor with her for three days, and the cord was wrapped around her neck so her heart rate and oxygen levels kept dipping.

We had seen so many specialists, and the main diagnoses were ADHD, learning disabilities, and sensory integration. Not one expert made the connection between her birth injury and her cognitive issues. After further examination, Dr. Harch told us that Emily also had a concussion, which she got from a car accident the prior August. This explained why her anger levels were so high. This had also been missed by the ER physicians.

After the first HBOT treatment, I could see a difference in her temperament. She was calmer than we had ever seen her. After two weeks of treatments, she texted her dad, and he wondered if Emily had actually written the texts. The logic, sentence structure, and spelling were so much better. At the end of the month, Emily told Dr. Harch, 'I can do math in my head now!'

I also decided to have the HBOT treatments while we were there. I had fallen off my bike onto cement when I was three and I got a concussion; I had another head injury when I was 10. In 2005, I slipped on black ice and hit my head yet again, which left me nonfunctioning. I was getting lost driving to work, I was exhausted, I couldn't sleep, and I couldn't add numbers, which is especially troubling because I am a financial auditor! Dr. Harch did a SPECT scan and said I would benefit from HBOT. I've had about 58 treatments altogether. My vision, sleep, energy, memory, and executive function all improved after treatments. The 'after' scans showed the difference.

I returned to New Orleans with our younger daughter, Sarah, who had been suffering from depression and anxiety for about three years. The doctors had diagnosed her with depression, which they said is typical for teenagers. She had counseling and medication, all with minimal results. Her depression was so bad that she stopped going to high school in the middle of her first year. She is a bright, athletic, capable girl who just tanked. So I faxed Sarah's records to Dr. Harch. Sarah thought she might have a brain tumor. He did SPECT scans and said, 'This is not the brain of a healthy 17-year-old.'

Sarah's left frontal lobe was about half the size of her right. This would explain the emotional swings, lack of impulse control, and poor judgment. Dr. Harch said the H1N1 virus (swine flu) she had in 2010 had damaged her brain. This was the reason she did not respond well to the protocol in Maine, which treated her symptoms and not the cause! Sarah also responded amazingly well to the HBOT and was back to her normal, happy self again.

Last winter, my husband took a leave of absence from work to bring Emily back down. Again, we saw great improvement with her from an additional 14 HBOT treatments. Her motor skills, thought process, decision making, and emotional responses have all improved. Dr. Harch told us Sarah would need another round. When Dr. Harch went over her SPECT scans, the changes were clear. Even a layperson like me could see the amazing results. She's now a freshman at the

University of Maine, and we plan to get some booster treatments at the end of the semester.

At first our insurance wouldn't pay for the treatments and we considered selling our house because we knew it would change our lives. There's research now that shows how HBOT helps within five years of an injury, so our insurance finally accepted our appeals and paid for all of our treatments after we submitted documentation. I tell people to get a referral for HBOT before going and to keep all your records and test results. I did research on this like I was back in graduate school. If you need help with your insurance company, I recommend contacting Laurie Todd, who calls herself 'the Insurance Warrior' (see the Resources chapter). She helps people negotiate appeals with insurance companies that refuse to pay claims.

I don't know where our family would be had we not made a huge leap of faith and done the HBOT treatments. We are so hopeful and thankful for what our children's futures will be."

What Are Concussions?

We now understand that, when left undetected, concussions can result in long-term brain damage and may even prove fatal. Surveys from the Centers for Disease Control and Prevention

(CDC) concur that the number of reported concussions has doubled in the last 10 years. Likewise, the American Academy of Pediatrics has reported emergency room visits for concussions in children ages 8 to 13 years old has doubled, and concussions have risen 200 percent among teens ages 14 to 19 in the last decade. Statistics also show that concussions caused by contact sports are a fast growing epidemic among both amateur and professional athletes

Did you know that your brain has the consistency of gelatin? It is cushioned from everyday jolts and bumps by cerebrospinal fluid inside your skull. But a violent blow to your head and neck or upper body can cause your brain to slide back and forth forcefully against the inner walls of your skull. This can affect brain function, usually for a brief period, resulting in signs and symptoms of a concussion. A brain injury of this kind may lead to bleeding in or around your brain, causing symptoms such as prolonged drowsiness and confusion that may develop immediately or later. Bleeding in your brain can be fatal. This is why anyone who experiences a brain trauma needs monitoring in the hours afterward and emergency care if symptoms worsen.[2]

Judith Kenyon's Story: Concussion

"I was at happy hour with friends in August 2015 when the ceiling of the century-old restaurant came crashing down and I was hit in the head with a piece of plaster. EMS came and asked me questions to make sure I was mentally competent. I wasn't unconscious, but I had a four-inch gash over my frontal lobe and I was in shock. I got a CT scan, which turned out to be OK, but an MRI showed damage to my brain.

Within the first week of the accident, I became seriously depressed and I completely withdrew. I would wake up in the morning feeling sad. I'm normally outgoing, happy, and extremely social. I even cancelled my trip to Santa Fe that I look forward to every year because I didn't feel like going. I went to my niece's wedding and I just sat in my chair and didn't talk to anyone.

My friends said 'Where did J. W. go and who is this alien that has invaded her body?' I found I was getting angry at people. I have a boyfriend who I've been with for 17 years and he was really worried about me. He said I needed to see a neurologist.

The neurologist diagnosed me with postconcussion syndrome. It's similar to what happens to football players. I didn't relate the depression with the hit on the head, but the doctor explained that the frontal lobe controls your moods and emotions. The neurologist sent me to a neuropsychologist where I got two days of intense testing. She said I had a traumatic brain injury.

This doctor and I had gone to Tulane together, and she said that my IQ had tested average even though she remembered me as a straight-A student. I was so despondent by this news. She told me she was doing a research project with Dr. Paul Harch and thought HBOT would really help me.

That's when my recovery began. Dr. Harch gave me a SPECT scan and recommended 40 treatments. After the first session I went home with my sister and I felt completely different. I was socializing again. My sister said, 'You've only had one treatment and I feel like I'm getting my sister back!' The SPECT scan after one treatment showed some areas of my brain that were previously dark were now lit up. The blood flow was coming back. I felt so much better. I've gone for HBOT every day since January and I've had 39 treatments— only one more left. I'm now feeling better than ever and I'm even starting to remember things I'd forgotten from my childhood. I know HBOT is rooted in science, but to me, it's like a miracle!"

Hail Mary for HBOT as Concussion Treatment

Football Hall-of-Famer Joe Namath discovered the benefits of treating concussions with hyperbaric oxygen therapy. Namath, who has

taken his fair share of sacks, was so pleased
with the results that he formed the Joe Namath
Neurological Research Center in Jupiter, Florida, to further the research of HBOT in cases of
TBI. Thanks, Broadway Joe!

Chris Borland's Cautionary Decision

It was "minor concussion" that got Chris Borland thinking
that playing football might not be worth the millions that come
with being a National Football League (NFL) player. Borland
was a rookie linebacker in his first training camp when he got
his "bell rung," he told ESPN's "Outside the Lines."

He kept playing and had an excellent rookie season. But
he worried that he might have sustained permanent brain
damage, so he spoke to his teammates and family and read
about the long-term effects of concussions. He ultimately decided to retire from football at the age of 24.

"I just honestly want to do what's best for my health," he
told ESPN. "From what I've researched and what I've experienced, I don't think it's worth the risk . . . I'm concerned that if
you wait [until] you have symptoms, it's too late." Borland, a
third-round pick from Wisconsin, turned his back on a $3 mil-
lion contract for four seasons with the San Francisco 49ers.

Borland is one of the first football players to retire before concussions became a health concern, but he is part
of a movement in sports that culminated with thousands of

former NFL players and their families cutting a deal in a 2015 class-action suit that called for the NFL to cover the cost of concussion-related head injuries. Reports show that an increasing number of retired NFL players who have had concussions suffer from memory and cognitive loss, dementia, Alzheimer's, depression, and CTE.

The suit alleged that the NFL deliberately misled players about scientific data that the medical community had found about the risks associated with concussions. In July 2014, a federal judge granted preliminary approval to the landmark deal, but the case is pending appeals at this writing. Chris Dronett was one of the plaintiffs. Her husband, former Denver Bronco Shane Dronett, committed suicide in 2009 when he was 38. After his death, an autopsy revealed evidence of CTE in his brain.

This controversy was the subject of a 2015 feature film *Concussion* starring Will Smith, who played Dr. Bennet Omalu, a Nigerian forensic pathologist who fights against efforts by the NFL to suppress his research on CTE suffered by professional football players.

"I've thought about what I could accomplish in football," Borland said, "but for me personally, to be the type of player I want to be in football, I'd have to take on some risks that I don't want to take on."

Michel and Mathieu's Story: Cerebral Palsy

Thomas Fox, a member of the American Association for Hyperbaric Awareness, has a master's in aeronautical science and psychology. He is a certified HBOT practitioner who lives and works in Montreal, Canada. His passion for HBOT is personal as well as professional. He is the stepfather of two boys born at 27 weeks with cerebral palsy. This is his story.

"My two stepsons, Michel and Mathieu, survived a condition called twin-to-twin transfusion, where one twin has too much blood and the other doesn't have enough. In 1997, when they were four years old my wife, Claudine, took them to England for treatment after doing research on cerebral palsy treatments to reduce their spasticity (a condition in which certain muscles are continuously contracted). England had a network of chambers used to treat multiple sclerosis. I met my wife at a conference there where she was speaking about the topic.

Both boys were in wheelchairs at the time. Michel couldn't open his hands or speak. After 24 treatments, Mathieu was out of the wheelchair and Michel was talking. The Canadian Broadcast Company and Canada TV followed their stories, which helped raise funds for their treatments. The headline was 'Mother Takes Children to England for Experimental Treatment.' The boys were filmed going onto the plane in wheelchairs and then running off the plane after HBOT treatments. Now they're 21, and they can give media interviews in both French and English.

Mathieu has had total recovery except for a limp. Michel has some learning issues, but he can take care of himself, do laundry, and cook. He's living at home with us now, but he wants to get his own apartment. All told, they've had 950 treatments and they are continuing to show improvements."

Elizabeth Hardy's Story: Autism

"I'm the mom of Chase, who is eight, and Caleb, who is two. Caleb is my biological son. We were told that he has severe autism and that he would probably never speak. There are a few therapies out there, we were told, but this is your life—sorry.

When I heard about HBOT, I was intrigued. So we started going to conferences and doing as much research as we could. When Caleb was in preschool, we decided to try it. We rented a chamber and he did 40 dives. HBOT helped Caleb come out of his shell. If you met him today, you'd just think he was a quirky kid. He's now mainstreamed in second grade. He skis and plays other sports. The doctor who told me we'd never be able to fix this has a son in Caleb's second-grade class. We were told, 'Your child will never talk,' and now he can't stop talking! It makes me choke up just thinking about how well he's doing, but they are tears of joy—we are so grateful and happy to have him back."

Linda Small's Story: Autism

"My son, Sam, just turned 18. But I always knew something was wrong with Sam from an early age. He was verbal for a while but just stopped talking one day. I always read to him when he was young, but when he was about two, he would put his hand over his ears and over my mouth as if the sounds bothered him. He would never make direct eye contact. He would also have outbursts. If I didn't do certain things in the order he wanted them, he would have tantrums. I could push the stroller but my husband couldn't, for example. He would try to choke me when he got upset.

I kept asking his pediatrician what was wrong with him, but he didn't diagnose him. He said, 'I've heard him speak words to me—he seems just fine.' When I told him about the choking incident he said, 'Well, I think you've got to get a hold on him, maybe he needs a stronger hand.' This was a young doctor too.

So I started paying out of pocket to take him any place I thought could help him. I got him a hearing test. There wasn't anything wrong with his hearing, but at least the doctors could see that Sam had a problem. Instinctively I knew it was autism, but they were backlogged for years for testing. They told me to wait until he was in school so the school would be responsible for doing testing. By that time, he was a danger to himself.

Sam was completely nonverbal. He would bolt, and if he got away from me, he wouldn't be able to tell anyone his name. This was scary because I lived in a big city. I'd be holding his hand and he'd just run away. I made an oath then that I would find a new place to live. I owned a secretarial service in Tampa, Florida, which is where I met Dr. Maxfield. I was doing research for a customer and up popped the state of Vermont. I didn't even know where it was, but I believed that God was telling me to go there. Within a month, I bought a house there and we moved. I knew, if nothing else, the small community would come to know Sam, love him, and accept him, so even if he didn't get better, that's all I wanted.

When I moved to Vermont I was in for a culture shock. In my heart, I knew he had autism, but I still brought him to daycare every day. He didn't socialize and just sat in a corner, but I knew any contact with other children was good for him. In Vermont, people watch children out of their homes. I brought him to Head Start. I was blessed because when I took him to a pediatrician who was from Russia, she looked at him and asked, 'Do you think there's something wrong with your son?'

I said, 'Absolutely, I think he has autism, but no one will listen to me.'

She agreed with me and gave me an appointment with the state pediatrician, who diagnosed him with autism. After that he had a pathologist, physical therapist—anything we could want.

I had heard about hyperbaric treatments for autistic children through Dr. Maxfield and Dr. Neubauer. To be honest, I didn't have huge expectations. I was hoping for about a 1 percent improvement and came out of there with 100 percent belief in it. I took Sam to Florida for two weeks of HBOT. It made an amazing difference. Sam had always had short- and long-term memory deficits. I didn't tell his teachers that I was taking him for HBOT. When he returned to Head Start, he was ready to learn. He used to spend weeks relearning what he would lose over the summer. After HBOT, he started right where he left off.

Unfortunately, we couldn't afford to continue the HBOT treatments. Insurance won't cover this condition even though it opened up his neural pathways. It was cost prohibitive, especially after my husband developed cancer and hepatitis and lost his business. We never recovered financially because I had to cut back on my business to take care of Sam. At this point, I'm also disabled due to allergies that prevent me from going outside.

Sam is still in school and he is working as a dishwasher part time. He is going to the career center next year to take a computer class. He even has a girlfriend now who isn't on the spectrum. He can make eye contact, he can shake hands, and he can talk with people. He knows he's different, but he's able to deal with it. Academically he's on a sixth- or seventh-grade level. If the government would reverse its decision about HBOT, he would be able to do so much more. If you have an autistic child and you have the resources, you should absolutely seek out hyperbaric treatment."

What Causes Autism?

Not long ago, the answer to this question would have been "we have no idea," according to Autism Speaks, an

organization dedicated to increasing awareness and further-
ing research to improve the lives of those who struggle with
autism. Research is now delivering some answers. We now
know that there is no one cause of autism, just as there is
no single type of autism. Over the last five years, scientists
have identified rare gene changes, or mutations, associated
with autism. A small number of these are sufficient to cause
autism by themselves. Most cases of autism, however, appear
to be caused by a combination of autism risk genes and environmental factors influencing early brain development.

In the presence of a genetic predisposition to autism, a
number of nongenetic, or "environmental," stresses appear
to further increase a child's risk. The clearest evidence of
these autism risk factors involves events before and during
birth. They include advanced parental age at time of concep-
tion (both mother and father), maternal illness during preg-
nancy, and certain difficulties during birth, particularly those
involving periods of oxygen deprivation to the baby's brain.
Keep in mind that these factors by themselves do not cause
autism. There is a combination of factors that modestly increase risk, and there is no scientific evidence connecting
vaccinations to autism.

How Common Is Autism?

Autism statistics from the CDC identify around 1 in
68 American children as being on the autism spectrum.
Studies also show that autism is four to five times more
common among boys than girls. An estimated 1 out of 42
boys and 1 in 189 girls are diagnosed with autism in the

United States. Autism spectrum disorder affects over 3 million people in the United States and tens of millions worldwide. Government autism statistics suggest that prevalence rates have increased 10 to 17 percent annually in recent years. This increase might be due to better awareness of the condition.[3]

8 BREATHE EASIER: PULMONARY CONDITIONS

. . . .

Oxygen and Stem Cells for Chronic Obstructive Pulmonary Disease

Chronic obstructive pulmonary disease (COPD) is an umbrella term used to describe progressive lung diseases, including emphysema, chronic bronchitis, refractory (nonreversible) asthma, and some forms of bronchiectasis, a condition where the bronchial tubes of your lungs are permanently damaged and enlarged. The disease typically develops in people who are 40 or older, and more than 24 million Americans have it, according to the COPD Foundation. Lung disease is also the third leading cause of death in the United States. COPD gradually makes it difficult for the sufferer to breathe. Cigarette smoking is the leading cause, but long-term exposure to lung irritants might also put you at risk.

Traditional treatments for COPD used in the last 30 years have proven to be ineffective. For this reason, many are now turning to HBOT for treatment. One of my patients with COPD came to me after visiting a major medical center in California. Doctors there gave her only a few months to live. She was beginning to lose cognitive function from oxygen deficiency. When we started her on HBOT, her symptoms reversed and she lived five more years before succumbing to other complications unrelated to COPD.

There has also been increasing acceptance recently of the value of regenerative medicine, including the use of stem cells. We now know that HBOT can significantly increase the availability of stem cells in a patient's body by a factor of approximately eight. In this way, hyperbaric oxygen is doing exactly the same thing as stem cell treatment for COPD and other lung conditions. According to the Lung Institute, 84 percent of people with COPD have benefited from stem cell treatment, thanks to the passage in 2015 of the Stem Cell Therapeutic and Research Reauthorization Act. This law will help provide funding for stem cell research in the next five years.

Even the Catholic Church has shown interest in regenerative medicine by holding the Third International Conference on Progress of Regenerative Medicine and Its Cultural Impact at the Vatican in April 2016. With the increasing interest in stem cell treatment and the recognition of how hyperbaric oxygen promotes the availability of stem cells in the body, my hope is that both stem cell therapy and HBOT will be used for more chronic diseases in the future. When we add stem cell therapy to the regenerative properties in hyperbaric oxygen therapy, the results are sure to be spectacular![1]

Alicia's Story: Emphysema

In 1995, a physician friend of mine installed a hyperbaric chamber in his home to treat his wife's emphysema. His wife, Alicia, later suffered a stroke that left her bedridden. She gradually lost a significant amount of weight (down to a mere 76 pounds), and she was put on supplemental oxygen. She suffered from dementia caused by lack of oxygen, and her doctors gave her only two to three months to live.

At that point, Dr. Neubauer and I stepped in, using her husband's chamber to administer hyperbaric oxygen. We started with very low pressure, and Alicia began to respond within weeks. Soon she no longer needed supplemental oxygen, her appetite improved, and she gained 36 pounds. She was once again back to her bright, active, energetic self and was no longer confined to her bed. Alicia lived another five years thanks to her daily hyperbaric oxygen treatments.

While HBOT is not a cure, in the same way that insulin does not cure diabetes, it can prolong and improve one's quality of life. This case confirms the findings from many studies about the remarkable benefits of HBOT in treating chronic pulmonary conditions.

Fiber for Better Breathing

Most people know about the enormous health benefits of fruits and veggies, whether they eat the recommended amount or not (adults should consume 1.5 to 2 cups of fruit and 2 to 3 cups of vegetables daily, according to the CDC). Most people don't come close to that. Here's some more motivation: A high-fiber diet, especially from plant-based foods, can protect you against such lung conditions such COPD and asthma. A recent study found that among more than 1,000 adults, those who ate the most fiber daily had the best lung function. Why? Inflammation underlies many lung diseases, and fiber has anti-inflammatory properties. Fiber also changes the composition of the gut microbiota (the good bacteria in our stomachs), which may release compounds that protect the lungs.[2]

Ruth's Story: Asthma and Allergies

Ruth is a British freelance writer who shares information about allergies, eczema, asthma, and food intolerances. Her website, www.whatallergy.com, was voted one of the top-five allergy blogs on the Internet. Here's what she had to say about her HBOT experience in one of her blog entries.

August 18, 2011

"Imagine a spaceship or a submarine with tiny round porthole windows. The chamber can seat about four to six people comfortably on padded chairs. Hyperbaric oxygen therapy has been around for a long time, originally invented to treat divers with the bends, the chambers are now widely used across the UK at local MS centers to treat, not just MS, but a wide range of other medical conditions and sports injuries. . . . To read more about studies which suggest oxygen therapy can indeed help alleviate allergies and even autism, see what Jane Dean has to say about 'Hyperbaric oxygen and inflammation—how it can also be used to treat allergy and, maybe, even autism' on the Foods Matter website.

For the first 10 minutes of the treatment you can chat and talk freely to other people in the chamber whilst the technician gets the chamber up to the correct pressure. Then the signal to don masks is given and we all put on our half face masks and settle in for the long haul.

You breathe 100 percent pure oxygen for an hour, during which time you can read, listen to music, play cards or just relax. I read a book and practiced some yogic breathing; I actually felt myself relaxing so much I almost put my head back and let my eyes close. I never sit down for an hour and just read or relax—so this forced inactivity was actually quite liberating. I really should take time out to meditate or just relax rather than rushing around all the time. It was incredibly relaxing. You become very aware of each breath in because you can hear it rushing through the mask. You can count how many seconds each breath takes, breathing in deeper and longer and experimenting with your breathing.

I might be imagining it, but along with an amazing sense of peace, calm and well-being I also feel like I'm breathing more freely, and cycled all the way home without once wanting or needing to use my inhaler. Just a coincidence? Impossible to see improvements in such a short time? Who knows? Perhaps I was just buzzing from the exhilaration of a bike ride in the English summer sunshine (where did that go?). What I do know is that I'm actually now feeling really positive, motivated and excited about where this treatment might take me."[3]

HBOT and Asthma

In addition to treating COPD, hyperbaric oxygen can stop an asthmatic attack, decreasing the need for steroids and hospitalizations. A young man who became a patient of mine was routinely admitted to the hospital after asthma attacks, sometimes as often as three times a year. After receiving HBOT treatments, he went for more than three years without needing steroids or being hospitalized. He also grew five inches during the time he was not taking the medication.

Just a one-dose pack of steroids can wipe out the blood supply to the growth centers in our body for up to one year, a nasty side effect when used by children who are still growing. This accounts for the short stature of asthmatic children and young people who have been on a course of steroids. Another complication of steroids is the risk of developing aseptic necrosis (the death of bone tissue due to a lack of blood supply) after only one dose of a steroid injection.

SEEING THE LIGHT: OPHTHALMOLOGY

A firefighter suffered cortical blindness after being struck by lightning during one of his rescues. Ophthalmologists who examined him were unanimous in their belief that his condition could not be cured, and his vision loss continued for three years after the incident. It wasn't until he saw Dr. Richard Neubauer, who gave him 20 hyperbaric treatments, that his vision was restored. After 40 HBOT sessions, the fireman's eyesight was better than it was prior to the lightning strike!

HBOT has also been found to work with congenital blindness and corneal ulcers and as an aid in treating diabetic retinitis and other ocular conditions, such as retinal detachment or blockages and even macular degeneration. Recent studies show evidence that an increase in oxygen can help improve vision in humans. It does so by affecting the inner and outer layers of the retina and by helping to normalize damaged retinal tissues.[1]

Nate's Story: Vision Loss

"I'm a Seattle-based registered nurse and mom of Nate, who is now 17 years old. When Nate was 10, he received a brain injury playing lacrosse. He had some severe aftereffects, including pain, balance problems, hearing, and cognitive function loss. His most serious problem was his eyesight. Nate's entire peripheral vision was knocked out by the injury—he could only see an inch in front of each eye with mostly clear sight—the rest of his vision was totally opaque and spinning constantly. The doctors determined the hit had knocked out his brain's ability to move his eyes from side to side. For a year and a half, we went to a slew of doctors, ophthalmologists, optometrists, neurologists, and other specialists. Eventually we went to a physician who is known as 'the god of eye doctors.' He actually told Nate that his vision would never improve.

As a registered nurse, I come from a conventional medical model, so it was natural for me to first seek intensive rehab and medical and pharmacological support. Over the course of the first year and a half after his injury, we were told that there was no cure for Nate's eyesight and that the only treatment was supportive care, rehab, and medications. Some of his symptoms did improve over time with these and other therapies, but his eyesight never improved.

I read over 500 medical journal articles about brain injuries and vision loss. I came across an article by Dr. Paul Harch in the *Journal of Neurotrauma* about the use of hyperbaric oxygen therapy in brain injuries. The results were extremely positive: not only did the post-brain-injured veterans self-report to being better and feeling better, but the SPECT scans of their brains confirmed improved oxygenation and circulation to the damaged parts of their brains.

I extensively researched both Dr. Harch and other practitioners of hyperbaric therapy, reading a multitude of national and international articles about the subject dating back 20 years. What I read convinced me that hyperbaric therapy was worth a try. Taking Nate to New Orleans from Seattle seemed like the only chance to improve his eyesight and other brain injury symptoms.

First we decided to check with Nate's Seattle physicians. They were almost universally opposed to the decision. They worried he would have seizures or even lose his eyesight all together. When I weighed their general input against the hard data and research I'd collected, it seemed clear their opposition was based not on the physics, medical science, or data on hyperbaric oxygen therapy in brain injuries but simply on lack of knowledge accompanied by some bias. These doctors had been willing to put Nate on multiple medications for life, many of which were considered off-label for brain injuries, but were not willing to consider a therapy that has been around many years and has minimal side effects.

Finally, I went to a neurologist who'd been a military doctor in Iraq and Afghanistan and had seen thousands of brain-injured veterans. He said if it were his boy, he'd try hyperbaric oxygen therapy. He told us, 'It's the only therapy that offers a hope for Nate. Why not try it?' So we did, even though, with a job, three other children, and elderly parents who need my help, it wasn't easy to travel across the country for medical treatment that would last five weeks. It is the best decision I ever made. Nate, who was so impaired that a therapist said he was the sensorial equivalent of a C1 quadriplegic, is now, after 80 hyperbaric treatments, 90 percent better. His physical mobility and balance are much improved, and his cognitive function is so much better that he is getting As and Bs in school! His unremitting headaches are gone, and his eyesight is dramatically better. He went from not being able to see the difference between a pickup truck and a compact car to being able to read the *Hunger Games* in regular print.

In Dr. Harch's waiting room, I saw many patients get much better, including a 10-month-old with cerebral palsy who'd been certified by several prominent ophthalmologists to be cortically blind. After hyperbaric therapy, this child was examined by those same doctors who said they'd never seen anything like it but confirmed that she'd regained all of her vision in one eye and the other was much improved. We are thankful we made the decision to ignore the naysayers and get Nate HBOT."[2]

Vivian Greene's Story: Vertigo

"I was in three car accidents during a six-month period while I was living in Hawaii in 2001. The first crash was a hit-and-run with a driver going the wrong way on a one-way street. In the second, I was rear-ended by a guy who was on his cell phone, and in the third, I wasn't driving but got hit on the passenger side after we pulled out of a driveway.

The first accident injured my neck and gave me vertigo. The dizziness was so bad that I would fall down a lot. I fell down once in my kitchen once and broke my arm. Doctors prescribed Dramamine, which is what you take if you're seasick. It would work for a few days and then the vertigo would come back. I had the vertigo for 10 years until I started doing hyperbaric oxygen therapy with Dr. Maxfield in 2015 after I tripped on a hole in the ground. After the HBOT treatments, the dizziness stopped.

After the accident, my leg became swollen and painful and my vision was affected. My depth perception was off, and I began bumping into walls and furniture. I went back for HBOT treatments, this time seven days a week, which brought the swelling in my leg down. After about 20 sessions, I was going to stop when I suddenly noticed that I had 20/20 vision! Things looked blurry when I put on my glasses. I went to my optometrist and he asked me if I had laser surgery. I told him it was the HBOT. He gave me an eye test and I could read the bottom line with no trouble! HBOT not only helped cure swollen leg, it improved my eyesight and vertigo! I hear there's an ophthalmologist in Florida who now has a hyperbaric oxygen chamber.

If that wasn't enough, there was one other unexpected benefit from hyperbaric oxygen therapy. People started telling me how good I looked. I said, 'What are you talking about I'm feeling terrible!' But sure enough, I looked in the mirror and the oxygen had taken some of wrinkles and lines on my face away. I'm 67 years old and people tell me I look much younger. I posted a video of myself on YouTube dancing after my hyperbaric treatments as a tribute to Dr. Maxfield. Now one of my favorite sayings is 'Life isn't about waiting for the storm to pass; it's about learning to dance in the rain.' And that's exactly what I'm doing!"

Caleb's Story: Febrile Seizure

"At 19 months my son, Caleb, had a febrile seizure [convulsions that occur in young children and are triggered by fever] at the hospital and he stopped breathing. Doctors were unable to revive him for 12 minutes. He suffered severe brain injury and he was not expected to live. After two weeks on a ventilator, they pulled out the breathing tube. He struggled to inhale, and we actually saw him die in our arms a second time. But he fought back and took a breath after 20 seconds and continued.

He was blind and deaf when we took him home from the hospital. We were told that he'd be in a vegetative state, that he wouldn't be aware of us, and that he'd probably die within two years from pneumonia. He was also spastic, with his arms locked over his chest. His legs were hyperextended and also locked. It took two of us to change his diaper and to give him his feedings. We gave him medications and took him to an acupuncturist. During the acupuncture, there was a doctor in another room being treated, and the acupuncturist told him about our situation. He said that we should get him immediately into hyperbaric treatments.

The following week, we started Caleb on a course of 40 HBOT sessions. After about 20 treatments, he began to relax a bit. When the 40 treatments were done, he could see again. After 160 dives, his spasticity reduced so we cut back on the medication. Caleb is now able to see, hear, and talk again. He's come so far and he's such a joy. Now we finally have hope!"[3]

10
BODY UNDER SIEGE: AUTOIMMUNE DISEASES

. . . .

On March 6, 1999, Shannon Kenitz gave birth to a beautiful baby girl named Grace. As happy as any parents would be to welcome another addition to their family, Shannon's joy began to fade as she noticed a drastic change in her child. Grace wasn't eating well and her eyes began to roll frequently. She was later diagnosed with a rare mitochondrial disorder and suffered repeated seizures. Mitochondrial diseases result from failures of the mitochondria, specialized compartments in every cell of the body except red blood cells. Mitochondria are responsible for creating more than

90 percent of the energy needed by the body to sustain life and support growth.

Diseases of the mitochondria, which primarily affect children, appear to cause the most damage to cells of the brain, heart, liver, skeletal muscles, kidney, and endocrine and respiratory systems. Shannon visited many physicians and explored various therapies, but Grace's condition turned life threatening. She was put on a feeding tube, she lost her vision, she was unable to walk, and she was on 42 different medications. Shannon and her eldest daughter, Lily, lived in a hospital for three years so they could monitor Grace's condition. The hospital eventually won the right to take Grace off of life support, and Shannon had exhausted all the insurance the state offered.

That's when Shannon heard about hyperbaric oxygen therapy through a national parent network for special needs children. After learning about the various benefits others experienced with HBOT, she immediately consulted Grace's pediatrician asking for a prescription. As is often the case, the doctor was unfamiliar with HBOT and wrote on his prescription pad: "Feed Grace with Styrofoam three times a day and she will get better." Shannon's disgust with her doctor fueled her obsession to get the therapy Grace so desperately needed. Thankfully, Shannon found another doctor who gave her a prescription for HBOT.

Shannon took Grace out of the hospital and drove her to Florida, where Grace would begin HBOT treatments. Miraculously, after 17 sessions Grace grabbed her mother's hand for the first time. She was finally showing improvement both physically and cognitively. As Shannon and her two daughters found themselves practically living full-time in another hospital, Shannon knew she had to go back home to save her marriage.

Four weeks after returning home to Wisconsin, Grace began sleeping 18 hours a day. Grace's brain was shutting down. Again, doctors were convinced that Grace would not survive. Shannon knew she had to bring HBOT to Wisconsin and ultimately to Grace. In just 12 weeks, she managed to get corporate sponsorship to open her own hyperbaric clinic in Madison, where Grace defied the odds yet again and regained neurological function.

Grace's story was the catalyst for Shannon to speak at medical and parent conferences to help inform other families with children suffering from similar conditions about the benefits of HBOT. Grace continued to progress. One day, Shannon was returning home from a conference and found herself greeted at the Madison airport by not only her family but also news cameras. To her amazement, Grace got out of her wheelchair and walked to her mother for the first time in her life, proving, once again, what HBOT can accomplish.

The remarkable recovery of her daughter led Shannon to become a spokeswoman for the International Hyperbarics Association. You can see and read more about her personal story and get information about HBOT at her website, www.shannonandgrace.com.[1]

What Is an Autoimmune Disease?

Autoimmune diseases affect up to 50 million Americans, according to the American Autoimmune Related Diseases Association.[2] An autoimmune disease develops when your immune system, which defends your body against disease, decides your healthy cells are foreign. As a result, your immune system attacks healthy cells. Depending on the type, an autoimmune disease can affect one or many different kinds of body tissue. It can also cause changes in organ function.

There are as many as 80 types of autoimmune diseases, including multiple sclerosis, lupus, type 1 diabetes, and celiac disease. Many of them have similar symptoms, which make them difficult to diagnose. It's also possible to have more than one at the same time. Autoimmune diseases usually fluctuate between periods of remission (little or no symptoms) and flare-ups (worsening symptoms). Currently, treatment for autoimmune diseases focuses on relieving symptoms because there is no curative therapy. You may be more susceptible to developing an autoimmune disease if you have a family member who has one.

What Causes the Immune System to Attack Healthy Cells?

The cause of autoimmune diseases is unknown. There are many theories about what triggers them, including

- bacteria or viruses
- drugs
- chemical irritants
- environmental irritants

What Are the Symptoms of an Autoimmune Disease?

Because there are so many different types of autoimmune diseases, the symptoms vary. Common symptoms include fatigue, fever, and just generally not feeling up to snuff. Symptoms worsen during flare-ups and lessen during remission. Autoimmune diseases affect many parts of the body, including

- joints
- muscles
- skin
- red blood cells
- blood vessels
- connective tissue
- endocrine glands (glands that secrete hormones)

How Are Autoimmune Diseases Diagnosed?

Ordinarily, your immune system produces antibodies (proteins that recognize and destroy specific substances) against harmful invaders in your body. These invaders include

- viruses
- bacteria
- parasites
- fungi

When you have an autoimmune disease, your body produces antibodies against some of your own tissues. Diagnosing an autoimmune disease involves identifying the antibodies that your body is producing.[3]

Multiple Sclerosis

One of the first doctors to use hyperbaric oxygen therapy to treat multiple sclerosis was Dr. Richard Neubauer, whose name has come up throughout this book. When my father-in-law began showing symptoms that included a loss of balance and deteriorating speech, my wife and I took him to four of the top neurological centers in the Southeast for evaluation. Not one was able to give him a definite diagnosis and they offered no treatment.

I had heard about Dr. Neubauer's excellent response in patients with multiple sclerosis (MS), so I took him to his HBOT center, even though I was unsure whether it would help. There, my father-in-law received a course of HBOT that kept his symptoms in check for three full years. At the time, which was the late '70s, it was customary to wait until symptoms recurred before providing additional treatment. Since then, patients with MS have shown that periodic HBOT sessions can provide better long-term results. My father-in-law might have had more good years had he received maintenance therapy, something that is now the accepted practice.

After meeting Dr. Neubauer, I began treating a number of patients with MS in my own practice at no charge, and I was pleased with the results. I joined the Gulf Coast chapter of the National Multiple Sclerosis Society, and I was elected chapter chairman in 1985. Unfortunately, the MS Society has yet to get on board with HBOT, so I was asked to step down as chairman after only one year. Despite the reluctance of the MS Society to accept any nontraditional or nonpharmaceutical treatments, I found HBOT continued to have excellent results with patients with MS. Although HBOT is not a cure for MS, it provides significant symptom relief and can delay or decrease the progression of the disease. I estimate the response rate for MS symptoms to be better than 80 percent, including increased mobility and strength.

The majority of neurologists whom I have worked with, however, did not agree with my assessment. One of my patients with MS could barely walk 60 feet from the parking lot into the office building prior to the HBOT treatments. After two months of hyperbaric oxygen therapy, she was walking two miles on the beach! Despite these amazing results, her neurologist reported "no improvement" because she still had a wide gait and some minor neurological symptoms. Despite this neurology report, she continued with her hyperbaric oxygen therapy and her condition remained stable.

Today, after more than 30 years of follow-up on two of my first patients with MS, one has only minor symptoms. The other, whose condition was more advanced, was told by her doctors that she would be bedridden within six months if she did not take her medication, methotrexate, a drug that is no longer recommended. She opted instead for using HBOT at my center and other "alternative" treatments. She was able to earn a doctorate, have two children, and continues to practice as a speech therapist despite being in wheelchair—much better than her initial prognosis.

In the many years that I've been using HBOT to treat MS, both for my own patients and as a consultant, I have yet to see any significant complications. There is a small risk of seizure, 1 per 10,000 dives, but these seizures do not produce long-term consequences and simply indicate the need to lower the oxygen pressure. Because of the great results with HBOT and patients with MS, some of the doctors who initially had a negative view of HBOT now serve as consultants in hyperbaric oxygen facilities.

Although insurance reimbursement for HBOT to treat MS is generally unavailable, a few of my patients have succeeded in getting coverage. Blue Cross Blue Shield of Texas paid for a monoplace chamber for one of my patients with MS, for example. With HBOT, she was able to resume her law practice and has had minimal progression of the disease. Another patient of mine had a complete reversal of MS symptoms after HBOT and sued Blue Cross Blue Shield of Florida for coverage. She was awarded full reimbursement plus payment for any additional HBOT treatments.

Similarly, one of Dr. Skaggs's first patients was a 38-year-old English teacher with MS from Arkansas. Her state did not allow doctors to perform HBOT treatments, so she traveled to Dr. Skaggs's clinic in Joplin, Missouri. She was an avid cross country runner before the onset. When she first arrived, she was, as Dr. Skaggs describes, "bouncing off the walls." She had cognitive function loss and she could barely walk. Ten treatments later, not only was she walking, but she also had no balance problems and got her memory back. After 20 additional treatments, she bought her own chamber, and now she's teaching again and running marathons.

Ella's Story: Lupus

Ella was 34 when she was diagnosed with lupus, a chronic autoimmune disease that can damage any part of the body (skin, joints, and/or internal organs). She developed osteomyelitis, a rare yet serious bacterial infection of the bone, in her finger. The condition got so bad that her doctors considered amputation. When called to consult on her treatment, I decided to add hyperbaric oxygen to her antibiotics. In 60 days, the osteomyelitis in her finger was cured by significantly increasing her hemoglobin, the protein molecule in red blood cells that carries oxygen from the lungs to the body's tissues.

HBOT and Crohn's Disease

You may have seen the commercials on TV promoting drugs for myriad ailments, including Crohn's disease, an inflammation of the small intestine. These ads are always accompanied by a long list of scary side effects. What you won't see in the media are promotions for safer, nonmedicinal treatments such as HBOT. I've had many patients with Crohn's disease who have made complete recoveries after hyperbaric therapy. The same has been the case for a similar condition called ulcerative colitis, which is an inflammation in the colon.

Unfortunately, because Crohn's disease and colitis are not approved indications for HBOT, they are not covered by insurance or Medicare. If you suffer from either of these conditions, I encourage you to seek HBOT treatments nonetheless. The day will come when both are approved for reimbursement, but until then, keep records of your progress with hyperbaric oxygen treatments and submit an appeal to your insurance provider. As I mentioned earlier, I have had patients who won their appeals with insurance companies by submitting documents that prove the efficacy of their HBOT.

HIV/AIDS and Hyperbaric Oxygen

An estimated 33.2 million people have lived with acquired immunodeficiency syndrome (AIDS) worldwide. People with AIDS have low blood oxygenation levels in addition to a damaged immune system, making them extremely susceptible to infection.

Because hyperbaric oxygen therapy increases oxygen levels in the blood, fluid, and tissues, it makes sense that this treatment can have numerous benefits for patients suffering from HIV/AIDS. Patients who reported debilitating fatigue showed relief within a month of receiving HBOT. I encourage anyone who has been diagnosed with HIV to get HBOT as soon as possible to reduce the virus in the bloodstream and decrease the damage in the small blood vessels that occurs as the initial infection spreads through the body. Of course, one should always consult with a physician before or during any kind of therapy for HIV/AIDS.

Austin and Sydney Williams's Story: Mitochondrial Disease

According to a 2011 article in the *Peoria Journal Star*, Scott and Gerri Williams were in a state of desperation when they brought their two young children, Austin, then 10, and Sydney, age 8, to see Dr. Zahangir Khaled at his pediatric gastroenterology practice in Peoria, Illinois. Dr. Khaled was the fourth specialist they had seen. "Austin and Sydney had been typical, non-complicated pregnancies," Gerri told the reporter. "But when Austin was 1 year old, he started regressing."

The Springfield-based mom quit her job as a registered nurse to care for her children full time. They had been sick for long periods of time and regressing physically and academically. Every doctor they saw, and they consulted many, was unable to pinpoint a diagnosis.

Dr. Khaled prescribed antibiotic supplements for the children to improve the beneficial bacteria in their digestive tracts. Next, he started them on an elimination diet, reducing foods that might be causing allergic reactions. Their condition did not change.

The family finally ended up at the Cleveland Clinic in Ohio, where the kids were diagnosed with mitochondrial disease, the same condition that Grace, Shannon Kenitz's daughter, suffered from.

"We were told that most children with mitochondrial disease don't live past 10," Gerri said, explaining that the disease prevents cells from using food to generate the energy needed to sustain life.

The children continued their steady stream in and out of hospitals as their health deteriorated. At one point, doctors discussed putting them on a ventilator to help them breathe, as well as a feeding tube so that their malnourished bodies could get some much-needed nutrients. Sydney was vomiting constantly and losing her hair. Both children had continual illnesses ranging from gastrointestinal upsets to ear infections, eye infections, and sinusitis. Austin was having seizures. Sydney had pneumonia three times in six months.

Gerri spent hours searching the Internet for clues to what appeared to be gradually killing her children. It was there that she found a glimmer of hope when she read about HBOT. "I was worried about talking to Dr. Khaled about it. I didn't know how he would respond."

But Dr. Khaled encouraged the parents to seek out hyperbaric treatment at the Wisconsin Integrated Hyperbaric Center outside Madison. There they were given four weeks of one-hour daily hyperbaric oxygen dives. Unfortunately, insurance did not cover these treatments, which cost over $7,000.

After just three treatments, however, the Williams family was stunned by the results. Back at their hotel, the siblings, who were normally low in energy, began shoving one another. "After the third treatment, Sydney was hungry. She gobbled lunch like she had never eaten before. She used to wake up at night screaming with stomach pain and throwing up. She also slept through the night," Gerri recalled.

The family's church collected $25,000 to buy a soft oxygen chamber that the Williams could use at home. After that, the kids got three treatments a week. They were weaned off nearly all their meds, and their health continued to improve. "Our children have learned to play like normal kids," Scott said. Their backyard now has a swing set and climbing beams, something previously thought impossible given the children's fatigue.

Dr. Khaled, who still sees Sydney and Austin, recommends HBOT to other patients with mitochondrial disease and hopes their amazing improvement will make more hyperbaric therapy clinics available to those with the disease.[4]

Sally Crawford's Story: Lyme Disease

"I didn't know that I had Lyme disease because I felt healthy and continued working and staying active until months after I was bitten by a tick. That's when I finally got a target rash and the disease brought me to my knees. Because I sought treatment so late, the antibiotics didn't work and only made my chronic Lyme condition worse. I saw many, many doctors who said they had never seen such a severe case as mine and told me there was nothing they could do. My organs were infected and were being ravished by the disease and I was told to get my affairs in order. I spent months in and out of hospitals getting treatments that didn't work.

While I was sick, I did tons of research, sometimes for eight hours a night, which was how I learned about hyperbaric oxygen therapy. I went to a clinic where I had nine months of HBOT treatments. It was a huge part of my recovery. HBOT kept me alive by supporting my organs and my body while I got detox and other treatments. It neutralized my infections, which allowed me to function again. I know the HBOT helped me because when I stopped for a day or two to help

take care of my father when he got cancer, my infection levels went up and I got really sick again. As soon
as I went back on the hyperbaric therapy, I was better.

Dr. Maxfield is brilliant, kind, and understanding.
He made sure I got the treatments I needed. Lyme
disease is different for every patient depending on the
bite and the level of infection in your body. If you catch
it early, you can be treated with antibiotics. The bulls-
eye rash only shows up in 50 percent of those who are
bitten.

I'm totally back to normal, and I'm back to work.
Without HBOT, I wouldn't be alive today."

About Lyme Disease

Lyme disease is a bacterial infection primarily transmitted
by deer ticks on the East Coast and black-legged ticks on the
West Coast. These ticks are typically found in wooded and
grassy areas. Lyme is found throughout the United States,
as well as in more than 60 other countries. It can affect any
organ of the body, including the brain and nervous system,
muscles and joints, and the heart.

The CDC estimates that 300,000 people are diagnosed
with Lyme disease in the United States every year. That's
1.5 times the number of women diagnosed with breast cancer and six times the number of people diagnosed with HIV/
AIDS each year in the United States. Because diagnosing
Lyme can be difficult, many people who actually have the
disease are misdiagnosed as chronic fatigue syndrome, fibromyalgia, multiple sclerosis, and various psychiatric illnesses.

The CDC notes that it is most common in children, older adults, and others such as firefighters and park rangers who spend time in outdoor activities and have higher exposure to ticks. Go to www.LymeDisease.org to see a symptom checklist to help document your exposure when seeing your health care provider.[5]

11

THE FUTURE OF HBOT

Perhaps sometime in the next decade, professors of medicine will have difficulty explaining why the treatment with (hyperbaric) oxygen was not widely adopted much earlier.

—Edward Teller, Nobel Prize–winning physicist

The more we learn about the life-changing impact of HBOT, the better the chances that hyperbaric oxygen therapy will be prescribed in the United States and around the world. Given the increased use of PET scans, which allow doctors to check for diseases in the body, and SPECT scans that clearly document the improvements before and after HBOT, hyperbaric oxygen therapy is poised to be adopted by mainstream medicine in the near future. I have no doubt that it can and will help even more people than it does now in the following areas:

HIV/AIDS: Equine oxygen therapy has been routinely and successfully used in Russia to treat AIDS patients because the pneumonia in AIDS is the same strain that horses contract.

Intensive care for TBI and wounds: HBOT will become a large part of emergency room treatment for traumatic brain injuries and wound healing. The ability to treat acute brain injury and severe wounds is unparalleled in any field of medicine. Traditionally trained doctors are discovering that, when used soon after surgery, it can reduce or eliminate postoperative inflammation.

Stem cell therapy: One of the most exciting advances for hyperbaric medicine is with stem cell therapy. We know that HBOT by itself can increase the stem cell population, which I and many scientists believe is the reason for the accelerated healing process that occurs when using hyperbaric oxygen therapy. The increase in stem cells might also contribute to the benefits of HBOT and stem cell therapy in spinal cord injury patients, whom, in other countries, are reportedly walking after paraplegia. From the stem cell conferences that I've attended, an obstacle has been the low take of the implanted stem cells. By using HBOT, we can enhance the take of stem cells, which, along with the developing technology, will improve patient outcomes in the near future.

Cancer care: We can and should be using HBOT as an adjunct to other treatments in cancer care. The day might soon come when we can use HBOT as a preventive treatment for people with cancer.

Birth injuries: There is huge potential for hyperbaric therapy when treating neonatal injuries, including premature and blue babies (infants with a blue complexion caused by a lack of oxygen in the blood). Blue babies can be the result of a congenital defect of the heart or major blood vessels. HBOT is now being used in other countries for women who have had miscarriages. When put on HBOT during their third trimester, these miscarriage-prone women are developing and maintaining healthy fetuses. This treatment in humans is based on the use of HBOT in horses that have not had successful pregnancies.

Aging: As we age, many of us lose some of our brain reserve. There is scientific evidence that HBOT can help improve cognitive function in the elderly and, with treatment, hopefully keep people out of nursing homes. Some of the conditions associated with aging that HBOT can be used for include

- arthritis
- stroke
- wrinkles
- diminished eyesight
- hip replacements

- delayed bone healing
- congestive heart failure
- Parkinson's disease
- Alzheimer's disease
- dementia

Home chambers: New hard-sided chambers are being developed for home use that give higher but safe levels of oxygen, which will make HBOT more affordable for patients requiring maintenance. At the moment, soft chambers are available for home use, and as you have read, many use these as an alternative to clinics or hospitals. Nevertheless, you should always consult a certified HBOT professional before buying and using a chamber for home treatments.

Precision medicine: So-called precision medicine is a growing trend in which doctors make treatment decisions tailored to the individual patient in a way that has not been fully utilized in the past. This is done by collecting data on the effectiveness of treatment programs and taking extensive family histories to help prevent and predict diseases in some patients. With this data, doctors should be able to determine how effective drugs actually are. In fact, many drugs on the market are not nearly as effective for some people as the preliminary approval for the medication has indicated.

The National Institutes of Health website (www.nih
.gov) has more information about this new program. You might even decide to become a participant. The data collected from this program incorporates genetic testing into the evaluation of patients that can aid in the prevention of some diseases and help slow down its development.

Modern technology allows health care practitioners to perform genetic testing quickly and at a reasonable cost, and the more this is done, the lower prices will become. This technology will ultimately shift medical treatment decisions toward a more holistic approach.

Traditional medicine today tends to treat the symptoms rather than the underlying causes of those symptoms. Once you pinpoint the cause of a problem, you can eliminate the symptoms, which, in my experience and opinion, is a far more valuable and effective approach to medicine.

SOURCE NOTES

Chapter 1

1 http://www.ihausa.org/

2 Dr. Maxfield and https://www.sharecare
   .com/health/emphysema/what-is
   -emphysematous-bleb

3 https://www.medicare.gov/coverage/
   hyperbaric-oxygen-therapy.html

4 National Institutes of Health.

5 http://www.mayoclinic.org; http://www
   .emedicinehealth.com/ct_scan/article_em
   .htm

6   http://www.www.mayoclinic.org/tests
    -procedures/pet-scan/basics/definition/prc
    -20014301

7   http://www.swanleytherapycentre.org/
    researchlatest-news/articles/telegraph
    -02022015

Chapter 2

1   http://www.hbot.com/article/hbot-chronic
    -tbi-oxygen-pressure-and-gene-therapy
    #overlay-context=user

2   *Diabetes Care* 33.5 (2010 May): 1143–45. doi:
    10.2337/dc10-0393

3   http://www.webmd.com/a-to-z-guides/
    wound-care-10/relieving-wound-pain

Chapter 3

1   Alzheimer's Foundation, http://www
    .alzfdn.org.

2   Paul Harch, *The Oxygen Revolution*, p. 49;
    phone interview notes.

3   Health Radar article by Dr. Maxfield.

4   Waistline study, http://www.ncbi.nlm.nih
    .gov/pmc/articles/PMC3358415/; *Beautiful
    Brain, Beautiful You* by Marie Pasinski and
    Jodie Gould.

Chapter 4

1   http://www.HyperbaricMedicalAssociation
    .org

2   National Heart and Lung Association,
    https://www.nhlbi.nih.gov/health/health
    -topics/topics/af

Chapter 5

1   http://www.ncbi.nlm.nih.gov/pubmed/
    20562529

2   Kohshi, K., Beppu, T., Tanaka, K.,
    Ogawa, K., Inoue, O., Kukita, I., &
    Clarke, R. E., "Potential Roles of Hyperbaric
    Oxygenation in the Treatments of Brain
    Tumors," *Undersea and Hyperbaric Medical
    Society* 40.4 (2013 July/August): 351–62.

3   http://emedicine.medscape.com/article/
    1157533-overview

Chapter 6

1   Cerdá-Olmedo, G., Mena-Durán, A. V.,
    Monsalve, V., Oltra, E., "Identification of
    a MicroRNA Signature for the Diagnosis
    of Fibromyalgia," *PLOS ONE*, March 24,
    2015, http://journals.plos.org/plosone/
    article?id=10.1371/journal.pone.0121903

2   http://news.rice.edu/2015/06/02/
    hyperbaric-hope-for-fibromyalgia
    -sufferers-2/#sthash.CZZkeG9q.dpuf

Chapter 7

1 Epilepsy Foundation.

2 Mayo Clinic.

3 https://www.autismspeaks.org/what
   -autism

Chapter 8

1 Health Radar (April 2016), http://www
   .copdfoundation.org/

2 Hanson, C., *BottomLine Health* 30.4 (2016
   April).

3 http://whatallergy.com/2011-08/
   hyperbaric-oxygen-therapy-diary-day1

Chapter 9

1 http://link.springer.com/chapter/10.1007
   %2F978-88-470-2198-3_19#page-1

2 Excerpted with permission from http://
   www.hbot.com/news/post-concussion
   -syndrome-treatment-hbot-mother
   -mother-letter

3 http://shannonandgrace.com/testimonials
   .html

Chapter 10

1 Shannon Kenitz is a spokeswoman for
   http://www.IHAUSA.org. This
   excerpt is based on the post on

http://www.shannonandgrace.com with written permission granted.

2 American Autoimmune Related Diseases Association, https://www.aarda.org/ autoimmune-information/autoimmune -statistics

3 http://www.healthline.com/health/ autoimmune-disorders#Diagnosis5

4 Howard, C., "Under Pressure to Improve Their Health," *Peoria Journal Star*, Health section, January 12, 2011.

5 http://www.lymedisease.org

GLOSSARY

anaerobic—The ability to grow or thrive in the absence of molecular oxygen.

ascent—Movement in the direction of reduced pressure, whether simulated or due to actual elevation in water or air.

atmospheres absolute—The sum of barometric and hydrostatic pressures. This is the most commonly used measurement when dealing with HBOT and is commonly referred to as ATA.

bends—The commonly used term for any form of caisson disease, or decompression sickness. It is sometimes a fatal disorder that is marked by neuralgic pains (severe pain along a nerve), paralysis, and difficulty breathing and is caused by the release of gas bubbles in tissue upon too rapid a decrease in pressure after a stay in a compressed environment.

decompression sickness—See "bends."

dive—A slang term for a hyperbaric treatment. It is rooted in scuba diving medicine. It is similar to taking a scuba dive because, in both cases, you breathe air or oxygen under pressure. The only difference with HBOT is that the increase in pressure is caused not by water but by using an air compressor or oxygen tank that forces increased air or oxygen into the hyperbaric chamber.

embolism—Air or gas bubbles in the arterial (artery: a vessel conveying blood from the heart) system caused by gas or air passing into the pulmonary (lung) veins after rupture of the air cells of the lung.

hydrostatic—Relating to the pressure that liquids exert.

hyperbaric pressure—Pressures greater than atmospheric pressure.

ischemia—Local reduction of blood supply due to obstruction of inflow of arterial blood.

osteomyelitis—Inflammation of the marrow of the bone.

pressurize—To increase the internal pressure of a closed vessel.

treatment depth—The depth or pressure to which a patient is compressed for treatment.

*Glossary excerpted with permission from Johnson Medical Associates in Dallas, Texas.

RESOURCES

American Association for Hyperbaric Awareness (AAHA; www.hyperaware.org)

The AAHA is devoted to advancing the understanding of hyperbaric oxygen therapy by bringing together professionals and scientists of diverse backgrounds and encouraging research and the application of new scientific knowledge to develop improved disease treatments and cures. It provides professional development activities, information, and educational resources for the public as well as medical professionals about

the results and implications of the latest
hyperbaric research. The AAHA also encourages discussions on ethical issues relating
to hyperbaric medical research and informs
legislators and other policy makers about
new scientific developments in hyperbaric
medical research.

American College for Advancement in Medicine (ACAM; www.acam.org)

The American College for Advancement
in Medicine (ACAM) is a nonprofit organization dedicated to educating physicians
and other health care professionals on the
safe and effective application of integrative
medicine. ACAM's health care model focuses
on prevention of illness and strives for total
wellness. The website will help you locate a
provider who specializes in complementary
medicine.

Bcenter.com (www.Bcenter.com)

Bcenter is a nonprofit organization run by
founder and CEO Valerie Greene that sup-
ports stroke survivors, like herself, and their
families. Her site includes published studies

about HBOT and other treatments for stroke and a link for locating practitioners.

Florida Veterans Foundation (FVF; www.floridaveteransfoundation.org)

The FVF offers free HBOT treatments for qualifying veterans through the Choice Program, including travel and accommodations. To speak to someone about applying, call 850-488-4181.

HBOT Online (www.HBOT.com)

This website, created by Dr. Paul Harch, provides information and links to resources on a wide range of HBOT topics.

International Hyperbarics Association (IHA; www.ihausa.org)

The International Hyperbarics Association is an educational and charitable organization that focuses on the needs of the hyperbaric community. Members range from medical centers treating the hyperbaric needs of patients to individual hyperbaric chamber users. As a teaching institution, the IHA distributes and publishes data, articles, and papers about the latest hyperbaric news and strides. If you are in need of hyperbaric treatment and you can't afford it, contact the IHA to see if you qualify for a grant.

International Hyperbaric Medical Association (IHMA; www.hyperbaricmedicalassociation.org)

Dr. Paul Harch is one of the founders of this association, which was created to advance hyperbaric oxygen therapy across the entire spectrum of medicine. The site provides the latest information about HBOT, resources for patients and medical professionals and links to other information for finding treatment for you or a loved one.

Laurie Todd (The Insurance Warrior; www.theinsurancewarrior.com)

Todd has dedicated her life to helping people win appeals with insurance companies that refuse to pay claims. She's written two books that will explain how to research and write your appeal and then deliver it to the highest-level decision makers at your insurance company.

OxyHealth (www.oxyhealth.com)

OxyHealth provides safe, portable hyperbaric chambers to physicians, professional athletes, wellness centers, and families. All OxyHealth chambers are designed for patients to easily self-treat, which has fostered a cutting-edge trend in hyperbaric technology. Its portable line of cost-effective, easy-to-operate, and convenient chambers has been sold to hundreds of thousands of people worldwide. Note: Patients using home-based oxygen chambers should be under the supervision of a doctor or certified HBOT clinician.

Parent-to-Parent Network (http://www.p2pusa.org)

Parent-to-Parent builds a supportive network of families to reduce isolation and empower those who care for children with developmental disabilities or special health care needs and provides information on how to navigate and influence service systems and make informed decisions. Do a Google search to find a Parent-to-Parent network in your state.

The Brain Health and Healing Foundation (www.brainjury.org/blog)

Driven by the belief that more can be done for people who live with neurological conditions, the Brain Health and Healing Foundation

(BH²F), is a nonprofit organization that raises funds to advance unexplored research of innovative treatments for brain injuries and diseases that adversely affect millions of people.

Undersea and Hyperbaric Medical Society (UHMS; www.uhms.org)

The Undersea and Hyperbaric Medical Society is an international nonprofit association serving some 2,000 physicians, scientists, associates, and nurses from more than 50 countries in the fields of hyperbaric and dive medicine. UHMS provides an important source of scientific and medical information pertaining to hyperbaric medicine and diving through its bimonthly peer-reviewed journal, *Undersea and Hyperbaric Medicine*; symposia; workshops; books; and other publications. It organizes an annual scientific meeting at different US and international locations to permit review of the latest in research and treatments.

RECOMMENDED READING

Doc, I Want My Brain Back by Dan Greathouse
(Greathouse Books)

*Conquering Stroke: How I Fought My Way Back
and How You Can Too* by Valerie Greene (Wiley)

Hyperbaric Oxygen for Neurological Disorders by
John Zhang (Best Publishers)*Oxygen and the
Brain* by Philip B. James
(Best Publishing Company)

Oxygen to the Rescue by Pavel I. Yutsis
(Basic Health Books)

The Naked Mind by Sheldon F. Gottlieb
(Best Publishers)

The Oxygen Revolution by Paul G. Harch and
Virginia McCullough
(Hatherleigh Press)

SAMPLE HBOT STUDIES

Baugh, M. A. "HIV: Reactive Oxygen Species, Enveloped Viruses and Hyperbaric Oxygen." BaroAntiviral, San Diego, CA, September 2000, PubMed.

Boussi-Gross, R. et al. "Hyperbaric Oxygen Therapy Can Improve Post Concussion Syndrome Years after Mild Traumatic Brain Injury." *PLOS ONE*, November 2013.

Efrati, S., Fishlev, G., Bechor, Y., Volkov, O., Bergan, J., Kliakhandler, K., Kamiager, I., Gal, N., Friedman, M., Ben-Jacob, E., & Golan, H. "Hyperbaric Oxygen Induces Late Neuroplasticity In Post Stroke Patients—Randomized, Prospective Trial." *PLOS ONE* 8.1 (2013): e53716. doi: 10.1371/journal.pone.0053716. The current study aimed to evaluate whether increasing the level of dissolved oxygen by hyperbaric oxygen therapy (HBOT) could activate neuroplasticity in patients with chronic neurologic deficiencies due to stroke.

Figueroa, X. A., & Wright, J. K. "Hyperbaric Oxygen: B-Level Evidence in Mild Traumatic Brain Injury Clinical Trials." *Neurology*, August 2016.

Hoge, J. "The Ritual of Hyperbaric Oxygen and Lessons for Trx of Post Concussion Symptoms." *JAMA Internal Medicine*, November 20, 2014. Significant improvements in postconcussion symptoms and secondary outcomes, including posttraumatic stress disorder, depression, sleep quality, satisfaction with life, physical, cognitive, and emotional health function.

Hu, Q., Liang, X., Chen, D., Chen, Y., Doycheva, D., Tang, J., Tang, J., & Zhang, J. "Delayed Hyperbaric Oxygen Therapy Promotes Neurogenesis through Reactive Oxygen Species/Hypoxia-Inducible Factor-1α/β-Catenin Pathway in Middle Cerebral Artery Occlusion Rats." *Stroke* 45.6 (2014, June):1807–14. doi: 10.1161/STROKEAHA.114.005116.

Lee, Y. S., Chio, C. C., Chang, C. P., Wang, L. C., Chiang, P. M., Niu, K. C., Tsai, K. J. "Long Course Hyperbaric Oxygen Stimulates Neurogenesis and Attenuates Inflammation after Ischemic Stroke." *Mediators of Inflammation*, vol. 2013 (2013). Several studies have provided evidence with regard to the neuroprotection benefits of hyperbaric oxygen (HBO) therapy in cases of stroke, and HBO also promotes bone marrow stem cells (BMSCs) proliferation and mobilization.

Miller, R. S., et al. "Effects of Hyperbaric Oxygen on Symptoms and QOL of Service Members with PPCS." *JAMA Internal Medicine*, November 17, 2015. Participants treated in oxygen chambers had significant improvement in postconcussion symptoms and secondary outcomes compared to the control group.

Neubauer, R. A., Neubauer, V., & Gottlieb, S. F. "The Controversy over Hyperbaric Oxygenation Therapy for Multiple Sclerosis." *Journal of American Physicians and Surgeons* 10.4 (2005): 112.

Neubauer, R. A., & Yutsis, P. I. "New Frontiers: Anti-Aging Properties of Hyperbaric Oxygen Therapy." *Townsend Letter for Doctors and Patients*, July 2009.

Neubauer, R., & Walker, M. "Hyperbaric Oxygen Therapy." *Townsend Letter for Doctors and Patients*, December 31, 1998: 66–70.

Reillo, M. R. "Hyperbaric Oxygen Therapy for the Treatment of Debilitating Fatigue Associated with HIV/AIDS." Maryland Medical Center, Bethesda, MD, July 1993, PubMed.

Riello, M. R., & Altieri, R. J. "HIV Antiviral Effects of Hyperbaric Oxygen Therapy." Lifeforce Hyperbaric Medical Clinic, Baltimore, MD, Jan 1996, PubMed.

Thom, S. R., Bhopale, V. M., Valazquez, O. C., Goldstein, L. J., Thom, L. H., & Buerk, D. G. "Stem Cell Mobilization by Hyperbaric

Oxygen." *American Journal of Physiology—Heart and Circulatory Physiology* 290.4: H1378–86.

Wolf, C., et al. "Impact of Hyperbaric Oxygen on Mild Traumatic Brain Injuries." *Neurotrauma,* November 2012. PCL-M composite scores and ImPACT revealed significant improvement. Average of 30 percent reduction in symptoms. Serious side effects extremely rare.

Zhang, T., et al. "Hyperbaric Oxygen Therapy Improves Neurogenesis and Brain Blood Supply in Piriform Cortex in Rats with Vascular Dementia." *Brain injury* 24.11 (2010): 1350–57.

DISCLAIMER

The ideas and suggestions contained in this book are not intended as a substitute for consulting with a physician. All matters regarding your health require medical supervision. Names of medications are typically followed by TM or ® symbols, but these symbols are not stated in this book. Some of the patients in this book have allowed their real names to be used. In the remainder of cases, the names of the patients have been changed.

INDEX

Claim Your Own FREE Heart Rate Monitor Watch Package Now!*

IN THIS PACKAGE, YOU WILL RECEIVE:

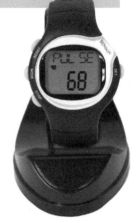

GIFT #1: Heart Rate Monitor Watch
With Easy-To-Read Instructions
(*A $49.95 value* — **FREE!**)

- Monitoring your heart by wearing a watch
- Tells you how many calories you burn
- Stop watch, daily alarm, and easy-to-see time and date

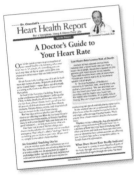

GIFT #2: Doctor's Guide to Your Heart Rate
An Exclusive Special Report (*A $15 value* — **FREE!**)

- Discover 6 simple ways to lower your heart rate
- How to know if you're getting the most from exercise
- How to determine your heart's "target zone," recovery rate, and safe maximum

GIFT #3: A Three-Month Trial Subscription
to Dr. Crandall's Heart Health Report
(*A $13.50 value* — **FREE!**)

Each month, you'll get incredibly important practical strategies to keep your heart running smoothly, including:

- How to lower you risk for a heart attack
- Keeping your blood pressure in check
- Easy ways to reduce your cholesterol level

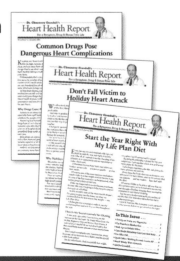

Go to: Newsmax.com/Watch411

*Just Pay $4.95 Shipping

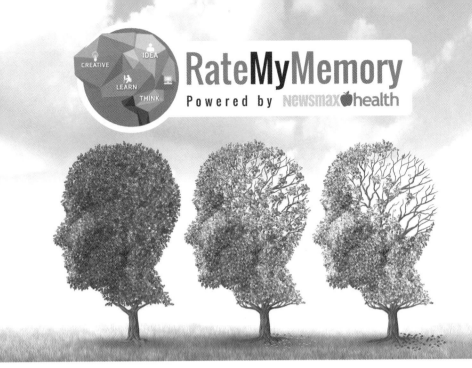

Is it Normal Forgetfulness?
Or Something More Serious?

You forget things — names of people, where you parked your car, the place you put an important document, and so much more. Some experts tell you to dismiss these episodes.

"Not so fast", says Dr. Gary Small, one of the nation's leading experts on brain health.

Dr. Small says that most age-related memory issues are normal but sometimes can be a warning sign of future cognitive decline.

Now Dr. Small has created the online RateMyMemory Test — allowing you to easily assess your memory strength in just a matter of minutes.

It's time to begin your journey of making sure your brain stays healthy and young!

Test Your Memory Today:

MemoryRate.com/HealthyTest